THE STRANGE CASE

OF THE WALKING CORPSE

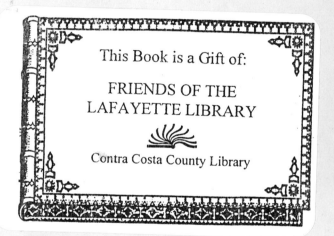

NANCY BUTCHER

THE STRANGE CASE
OF THE WALKING CORPSE

A Chronicle of Medical Mysteries, Curious Remedies,
and Bizarre but True Healing Folklore

AVERY • A MEMBER OF PENGUIN GROUP (USA) INC. • NEW YORK

Neither the publisher nor the author is engaged in rendering professional advice or services to the individual reader. The ideas, procedures, and suggestions contained in this book are not intended as a substitute for consulting with your physician. All matters regarding health require medical supervision. Neither the author nor the publisher shall be liable or responsible for any loss, injury, or damage allegedly arising from any information or suggestion in this book. The opinions expressed in this book represent the personal views of the author and not of the publisher.

The author has made every effort to provide accurate telephone numbers and Internet addresses at the time of publication. However, neither the publisher nor the author assumes any responsibility for errors, or for changes that occur after publication.

Most Avery books are available at special quantity discounts for bulk purchase for sales promotions, premiums, fund-raising, and educational needs. Special books or book excerpts also can be created to fit specific needs. For details, write Penguin Group (USA) Inc. Special Markets, 375 Hudson Street, New York, NY 10014.

a member of
Penguin Group (USA) Inc.
375 Hudson Street
New York, NY 10014
www.penguin.com

The images in this book are reprinted courtesy of the National Library of Medicine.

The poem on page 31 is from *The Essential Bashō*, translated by Sam Hamill. Reprinted by arrangement with Shambhala Publications, Inc., Boston. www.Shambhala.com.

Library of Congress Cataloging-in-Publication Data

Butcher, Nancy.
    The strange case of the walking corpse : a chronicle of medical mysteries, curious remedies,
    and bizarre but true healing folklore / Nancy Butcher.
        p.   cm.
    Includes bibliographical references and index.
    ISBN 1-58333-160-3
        1. Medicine—Anecdotes.   2. Medicine—Humor.
    3. Medicine—Miscellanea.   I. Title.
    R705.B88   2003   2003050244
    610—dc21

Printed in the United States of America
10   9   8   7   6   5   4   3   2   1

BOOK DESIGN BY MEIGHAN CAVANAUGH

Acknowledgments

Thank you to everyone who helped turn this idea into a book, including Laura Shepherd and Ken Siman. I want to extend an extra special thank-you to my editor, Kristen Jennings, for her patience, hard work, and insightful editing. As always, I am grateful to Jens David Ohlin for his unwavering love and support. He makes it possible for me to write and stay sane (well, relatively speaking, anyway).

In memory of my grandfather,

Dr. Hiroshi Sakata

CONTENTS

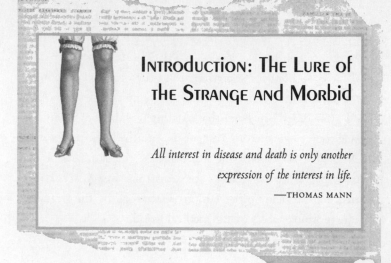

Introduction: The Lure of the Strange and Morbid

All interest in disease and death is only another expression of the interest in life.

—THOMAS MANN

THE SMELL OF FORMALDEHYDE

My fascination with medicine began when I was a young girl in Tokyo, where my grandfather Hiroshi Sakata was a doctor. He ran a small private hospital surrounded by a moat. I spent hours wandering around in his medical laboratory, peering into test tubes, staring at surgical instruments, perversely enjoying the smell of formaldehyde and other chemicals that lingered in the air. I know this was probably not a common preoccupation of young girls. But the truth was, I found petri dishes and pickled organ specimens much more engaging than Barbies and *Johnny Socko* episodes.

In high school, I excelled at biology and considered following in my grandfather's footsteps, until I realized that I would have to operate on cadavers—dead human bodies—in medical school. Since I could barely stomach dissecting frogs in biology class—I would always name them first, then weep while I sliced into their little green legs—I decided to pass on a medical career and opt for something less gruesome and corporeal.

Still, my interest in medicine never completely left me. And as I grew older I realized that this interest did not lie in the usual topics like anatomy, diagnosis, and the latest antibiotics (although I *did* ask for the *Merck Manual*, the standard physician's diagnostic handbook, for Christmas one year). I was lured, like so many other curious spectators, by the stranger, more morbid aspects of the medical world.

THE BIZARRE SIDE OF MEDICINE

Since the dawn of history, humans have suffered from ailments with strange, mysterious, sometimes downright gross symptoms. Whether it's the longest tapeworm ever passed by a human being (anywhere from 37 feet to approximately 108 feet, depending on which homespun Web site you consult) or elephantiasis (the hideous enlargement of scrotums and other body parts caused by lymph node blockage) or a case of uncontrollable vomiting during sexual intercourse, such conditions are well outside the realm of "Take two aspirins and call me in the morning." And the more bizarre the ailment, the more interested those who aren't afflicted seem to be.

Admit it: You're one of those people who slow down to stare at a particularly gruesome car wreck. The twisted metal, the smell of smoke, the urgent caravan of emergency vehicles— it gives you a secret, ominous thrill. *That person is in really bad shape,* you think. *And I'm not.* Or maybe you're just curious to see what death and dismemberment look like.

This is not to accuse you of being an unfeeling sicko (although I myself have had those moments). It's human nature to want to stare (and stare and stare) at gross, sicko things. It's also human nature to be curious about death and all the steps leading up to it.

Do you love those open-heart-surgery scenes in *ER?* Do you find those freshly dead corpses on *Six Feet Under* weirdly compelling? Do you savor those blow-by-blow descriptions of autopsies in Patricia Cornwell's mystery novels and find yourself wondering if you should have majored in forensic pathology instead of communications? Did you stare, transfixed, while Hannibal Lecter ravaged people's faces in *The Silence of the Lambs?* Then you're just like the rest of us.

The lure of the strange and morbid is a powerful thing. It's a way for us to look into the eyes of death—just for a brief second—and then look away. It's a way to feel more alive. It's a way to escape, even momentarily, from the sameness and smugness of our lives, and then retreat right back into them.

MEDICINE BY ANY OTHER NAME

Oftentimes, it isn't the disease that is so bizarre, but the cure. Unlike rare diseases, the treatment of common ailments and illnesses is something every person can relate to. At its best, medical practice consists of the skills of capable and committed doctors who cure our illnesses, medications that ease our symptoms with few side effects, and new technologies that reverse paralysis, heal damaged limbs, and perform a hundred other miraculous functions. At its worst, medicine fails us in both banal and tragic ways, from the annoyance of the common cold to a surgeon's inability to save a loved one on the operating table. People who have been failed by conventional medicine over the ages—or lacked access to doctors and medications—have sought remedies from unlikely, and even unsavory, sources. Snake venom injections, urine enemas, and the topical application of raw meat are just a few of the nontraditional cures that have been employed by the sickly, sometimes to disastrous effect.

Still, folk medicine—originating from the traditions and knowledge of common people—has been around for centuries. Way before med schools, the AMA, and HMOs, people relied on local lore, tribal knowledge, and/or religious tradition as sources of treatments to heal their ailments. After all, there was a time—and it wasn't so long ago—that it just wasn't possible to make an appointment with an ob-gyn or head over to the Rite Aid for a bottle of Advil.

Even now, folk medicine and its close relative, alternative medicine, thrive in the United States and other countries for a number of reasons. Some patients are dissatisfied with their experiences with conventional medicine: the side effects of procedures and medications, the dogmatic "doctor knows best" philosophy, and so on. Some patients have not found the cure or relief they're looking for, and turn to folk medicine as an alternative. Some believe that certain types of folk medicine are superior to conventional medicine. And some who suffer from an "incurable" chronic, debilitating, or terminal illness often turn to radical treatments in hope of a cure.

As time goes on, the lines between folk or alternative medicine and conventional medicine are getting blurrier. Cures that were once considered "the stuff of witchcraft" have become accepted by mainstream doctors. For example, the leaves and bark of the willow tree have been used since the time of the ancient Romans, often in tea form, to assuage pain and reduce fever. But now we know that willow trees and aspirin share a common ingredient.

While there can be antagonistic relationships between those who practice conventional medicine and those who practice folk or alternative medicine ("You're a bunch of wackos" versus "All you care about are freebies from pharmaceutical reps"), there can be symbiosis as well. Different practitioners from different schools of thought can learn from each other's successes and mistakes. Well-regarded medical journals publish articles on acupuncture and other treatments that were once considered solely alternative as more patients turn to these therapies for treatment

Also, we know that wonderful new discoveries sometimes can come from wild improvisation or even by sheer accident. For example, the antimalarial drug quinine was discovered quite by chance—or so goes one popular account. According to Lexi Krock in her *Nova Online* article "Accidental Discoveries":

> The story behind the chance discovery of the antimalarial drug quinine may be more legend than fact, but it is nevertheless a story worthy of note. The account that has gained the most currency credits a South American Indian with being the first to find a medical application for quinine. According to legend, the man unwittingly ingested quinine

while suffering a malarial fever in a jungle high in the Andes. Needing desperately to quench his thirst, he drank his fill from a small, bitter-tasting pool of water. Nearby stood one or more varieties of cinchona, which grows from Colombia to Bolivia on humid slopes above 5,000 feet. The bark of the cinchona, which the indigenous people knew as *quina-quina*, was thought to be poisonous. But when this man's fever miraculously abated, he brought news of the medicinal tree back to his tribe, which began to use its bark to treat malaria. Since the first officially noted use of quinine to fight malaria occurred in a community of Jesuit missionaries in Lima, Peru, in 1630, historians have surmised that Indian tribes taught the missionaries how to extract the chemical quinine from cinchona bark.

Today, quinine-based medicines are still used to inhibit the growth and reproduction of malarial parasites.

MEDICINE YESTERDAY, TODAY, AND TOMORROW

History is full of tales of medical curiosities: bizarre remedies, intrepid but foolish doctors, gross-out diseases, and more. Lest you think that all the strangest, weirdest, most interesting stuff in the world of medicine happened in the "olden days," prepare to be enlightened! Modern medicine, including modern folk medicine, is rife with stories of odd ailments and even odder remedies. Operating rooms and hospital wards are full of "procedures gone wrong" and other bad happenings.

And the medicine of tomorrow is even more fascinating. As I write this, our brilliant scientists are busily cranking out technologies that will enable us to regenerate limbs and organs, live to be 150, and allow ourselves to be cloned.

In writing this book, I have attempted to collect some unusual medical anecdotes, facts, and cures from the time of the ancient Greek physician Hippocrates to today. I did my research in a variety of places: medical journals, books, magazines, newspapers, and elsewhere. I have cited the sources where appropriate and available in the bibliography. In cases where anonymity was important, names and other details have been changed to protect privacy.

The Web was a particularly rich source of information. With our growing, aging population, there are hundreds if not thousands of Web sites devoted to medicine and health. Some are fairly conventional, standard, and reliable sources for medical information. Some are, to put it mildly, "really out there," with graphic personal descriptions of diseases and symptoms, adventures with experimental cures, and suggestions for . . . well, really bizarre-sounding treatments that involve animal parts, bodily waste, poisonous herbs, chants, and more. Much of this latter category provided content that is probably more entertaining than accurate.

Here are a few final points that merit a mention:

- If you suffer from an illness or have undergone a procedure or treatment mentioned in this book, I hope you will not take offense. This book is not meant to make light of the suffering of others. It is meant to *shed* light on areas of medicine not commonly known to laypeople. I have great respect for the terrible and terrifying powers of death and disease, which is part of the reason I wrote this book: It is my feeble attempt to tame the untamable.

- Unless you are particularly strong of stomach, you probably don't want to read this book before, during, or after a rich meal. And if you are prone to bad dreams, you would do well to avoid this book before bedtime.

- Except for the list of common home remedies on pages 65–67, **PLEASE DO NOT TRY ANY OF THE TREATMENTS AT HOME.** Neither my publisher nor I wish to receive a letter from you asking us why your arthritis symptoms didn't improve, and why you developed a strange green glow, after you sat in an abandoned uranium mine for many hours (a dangerous and unproven folk remedy for arthritis).

That said, I hope you will be as intrigued by these stories as I was while researching and writing this book.

A votre santé!

The Author

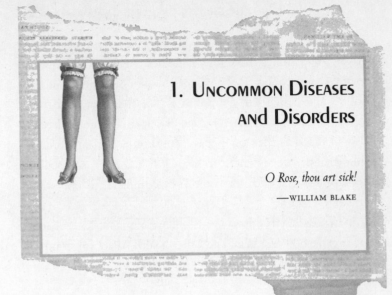

1. Uncommon Diseases and Disorders

O Rose, thou art sick!
—WILLIAM BLAKE

WHEN WE THINK OF MEDICAL DISEASES AND DISORDERS, we think of the usual suspects: heart disease, stroke, diabetes, hypertension, and the rest of the lot. Of course these illnesses are terrible and even life-threatening. But there are other illnesses out there—terrible and not so terrible, life-threatening and not so life-threatening—that many people have never heard of or know little about. This chapter will introduce you to a few of the strangest, grossest, or, in some cases, deadliest of them. Some of these ailments will disgust and terrify you. Some will strain your credulity and challenge your imagination as to what viruses, bacteria, and other undesirable agents can do to the human body.

I selected this list of unusual diseases and disorders for several reasons, since there are literally thousands of such diseases and disorders out there. Some have interesting historical aspects.

Some are really horrible ways to go. Some have spurred the use of radical, at times ridiculous remedies. And of course, as a writer, I must confess that some of the illnesses caught my eye not so much for their symptoms as for their nomenclature. Who says diseases can't have laugh-out-loud names? I have also included entries on bizarre conditions and anatomical abnormalities documented in historical literature. After all, a book on medical oddities wouldn't be complete without some "freaks of nature."

After reading this chapter, you will never again take functioning organs, boil-free skin, and other health basics for granted.

DISEASES THROUGHOUT HISTORY

With SARS, anthrax, the threat of smallpox, and the continuing AIDS crisis, it's hard to imagine living in a more frightening time and place than our own. But throughout the ages, there have been mysterious, incurable diseases and massive epidemics that make the twenty-first century seem relatively benign.

The most striking example of such a biomedical scourge is the plague. Leprosy and rabies are two diseases that are less deadly but nevertheless interesting and important in the history of public health.

THE BLACK DEATH

Ring around the rosies
A pocketful of posies

Ashes, ashes
We all fall down!

According to Professor Norman F. Cantor in his book *In the Wake of the Plague: The Black Death and the World It Made,* this charming and familiar children's rhyme may not actually be about rosies and posies. It may instead be about Europe's fourteenth-century Black Death plague epidemic.

Considered by some to be the greatest biomedical crisis in history, the plague killed tens of millions of people, wiping out entire towns, villages, and cities and devastating economic and social structures through death, poverty, and famine. The disease and the frantic search for a cure are evident in the writings, artwork, and music of the times and places in history that were affected. In Professor Kantor's view, folklore at least suggests that the lyrics of this English children's poem reflect the efforts desperate citizens took to keep the deadly disease away. These efforts included flowers and other folk remedies used to fight the disease, all of them in vain as the inevitable result was "ashes."

Plague is an infectious fever caused by the *Yersinia pestis* bacterium. The *Y. pestis* bacterium is carried by the rat flea, which generally lives on rodents. An infected rodent can pass the bacterium onto a human, after which point human-to-human transmission is possible in some (but not all) cases.

In humans, the *Y. pestis* bacterium manifests itself in three forms of plague: bubonic, pneumonic, and septicemic. With bubonic plague, there is a painful swelling of the lymph nodes, known as "buboes." Other symptoms include vomiting, sleeplessness, fever, chills, and constipation. The rat flea is the direct source of the infection; humans cannot pass the disease to one another. With pneumonic plague, the lungs are affected, resulting in a severe cough and shortness of breath as well as fever and chills. With septicemic plague, the bloodstream is so flooded with *Y. pestis* that the patient dies before either the bubonic or pneumonic forms of plague has a chance to set in— sometimes within twenty-four hours of onset. Even though the words *bubonic plague* may sound more ominous than the other two, the bubonic form of plague is usually least severe of the three. During the Black Death epidemic, both bubonic and pneumonic forms of the plague were at work.

In the Middle Ages, the causes of the plague were completely unknown and generated panic and hysteria in the regions it affected. The large-scale devastation caused many desperate communities in the Middle Ages to believe that the onset of the Black Death was God's punishment for man's sins.

Experts of that time also blamed unfavorable planetary alignments. According to Professor Kantor, a group of University of Paris professors was asked to research the source of the plague. The commission of professors concluded that the plague had been caused by the unfortunate alignment of Saturn in the house of Jupiter.

According to the Web site of medieval historian Professor E. L. Knox, there was no shortage of ideas about prevention and treatment of the plague. The flesh of poultry, waterfowl, pigs, old cattle, and fish was not to be eaten. Olive oil used in combination with food was thought to be "deadly." Nothing was to be cooked in rainwater. Sleep during daytime was discouraged, as were bathing and too much exercise.

In addition to God and astrology, there were a number of more earthly factors thought to cause the Black Death. Some experts believed that it was an airborne disease, possibly because of the terrible smells emanating from the dead and dying. In order to ward off the fatal vapors, citizens employed an early form of aromatherapy, burning a mixture of aromatic herbs, flowers, and other plants, including lemon leaves, rosemary, laurel, and pine. Many people also dipped their handkerchiefs in scented oils and covered their faces before going out. Doctors also ordered a near ban on bathing. It was feared that frequent bathing would allow pores to become open and admit the airborne disease.

According to Professor Kantor's book, windows were also kept closed and covered with heavy cloths so as to keep the pestilence out (similar to our modern-day duct tape!). But affluent Europeans were not content with common drapes. Instead, many of them commissioned tapestries from the finest tapestry makers in Belgium and northern France to prevent the plague from entering their homes. These wealthy clients ordered very large tapestries with elaborate scenes from popular romances woven into the cloth, perhaps to mask their morbid purpose.

So desperate were people for a cure against this horrific disease that they were willing to try anything, and there was no end to the creative remedies that were used. According to Professor Knox, many believed that loud sounds would ward off the disease, and towns would ring their church bells to drive away the plague.

A variety of herbal remedies was employed, mustard and garlic being two of the most popular curatives. Angelica was

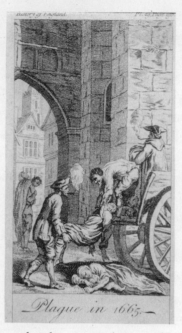

Plague in 1665.—

also used in accordance with a legend of the time in which an angel appeared to an afflicted peasant in a dream and revealed a cure that involved heating angelica over a fire with treacle and nutmeg. Local wise women and apothecaries offered other types of cures, charms, talismans, and spells, none of which worked.

There are some treatments from the Middle Ages that, though unsuccessful for treating the plague, are still used today as popular remedies. Barberry bark was taken with fennel seeds, probably in tea form, to prevent and treat the plague; it is used to this day by certain alternative health practitioners as an antiseptic, pain reliever, and laxative. In gem therapy, topaz stones, which were believed to have healing properties, were placed in water, which was believed to take on the supposed curative properties of the stones; it was then ingested as a medicine. Gem therapy is still widely practiced today for physical and spiritual healing.

Even in the Middle Ages, some people believed in the curative powers of positive thinking—especially against such a deadly disease with no known physical cure. One writer of the time advised that no one was to think of death; all thoughts were to be directed to happy, pleasant subjects. Walking through pretty, aromatic gardens and listening to beautiful music were activities to be encouraged.

In 1664 and 1665, the plague again brought chaos and calamity, this time upon the city of London. Masses of people died. Panic-stricken people tried to flee the city. Fires raged in the streets. Plague victims were shut up in their houses in an effort to prevent the spread of the disease. Cats and dogs were slaughtered, no doubt because they were thought to carry the disease.

Thomas Vincent, who survived the so-called Great Plague of London, wrote about the epidemic and its spiritual ramifications in a book (circa 1666) called *God's Terrible Voice in the City*. In it, he describes this scene:

> Now the citizens of London . . . begin to fear whom they converse withal and deal withal, lest they should have come out of infected places. Now roses and other sweet flowers wither in the gardens, are disregarded in the markets, and people dare not offer them to their noses lest with their sweet savour that which is infectious should be attracted. Rue and wormwood are taken into the hand, myrrh and zedoary into the mouth, and without some antidote few stir abroad in the morning. Now many houses are shut up where the plague comes and the inhabitants shut in, lest coming abroad they should spread the infection. It was very dismal to behold the red crosses, and read in great letters, "Lord, have mercy upon us," on the doors and, watchmen standing before them with halberts; and such a solitude about those places, and people passing by them so gin-

gerly and with such fearful looks, as if they had been lined with enemies in ambush that waited to destroy them.

The Great Plague of London killed 70,000 people—approximately 15 percent of the population. Two centuries later, in 1894, another epidemic sprouted in Canton and Hong Kong; over the next two decades, that epidemic killed more than ten million people around the world.

Just as the plague did not end with medieval Europe, it did not begin there, either. There are records in the Bible and elsewhere of apparent plague epidemics dating back many centuries before Christ. A particularly terrible epidemic struck the ancient lands in the Mediterranean around A.D. 540 during the reign of the Roman emperor Justinian. According to Dr. Frederick F. Cartwright in his book *Disease and History: The Influence of Disease in Shaping the Great Events of History:*

> The plague of Justinian may have been the most terrible that ever harrowed the world. We know something of it from the account written by Procopius, the secretary or archivist of Justinian's reign. It started in A.D. 540 at Pelusium in Lower Egypt, spreading throughout Egypt to Alexandria and to Palestine. Palestine seems to have been the focus of spread to the rest of the known world. It reached Byzantium in the spring of 542. The mortality was not at first great but rapidly rose until some 10,000 died each day. So many were the deaths that graves could not be dug sufficiently quickly. Roofs were taken off the towers of forts, the towers filled with corpses and the roofs replaced. Ships were loaded with the dead, rowed out to sea and abandoned.

Fortunately for many of us today, the plague is rare in developed countries. Isolated cases still occur today, however, usually in places with unsanitary, rat-infested conditions.

LEPROSY BY ANY OTHER NAME

Hansen's disease has been the official name for leprosy since the 1970s, in delayed acknowledgment of Gerhard Henrik Armauer Hansen, who diagnosed the illness in detail a century before. Hansen's disease is caused by the leprosy bacillus *Mycobacterium leprae* and is a chronic infection that damages the skin and nerves and causes disfigurement. Common symptoms include severely thickened and distorted facial skin and limbs. Eyebrows can fall off, and in serious cases extremities can fall off as well.

The route of infection is most likely via airborne droplets and skin contact; however, the disease is not easily transmitted from individual to individual unless they happen to live in prolonged, close contact. Antibiotics can improve the condition but not reverse or cure it.

For a long time leprosy was believed to be the result of some sort of curse. For this and other reasons having to do with fear of contagion, patients were ostracized and isolated in colonies. Leper colonies have a long, tainted, and tragic history: Victims were taken from their homes and families and shut away in isolated locations. Colonies still exist in the United States, on the tiny island of Molokai, in Hawaii; in India; in the Philippines; and elsewhere. In 2001 the government of Japan was sued by thousands of Hansen's disease victims who had been taken from their homes and incarcerated in a colony for many decades. The suit alleged systemic state discrimination and cruel treatment of patients, including forced sterilizations and abortions.

According to the Web site of Professor Arthur C. Gibson, who has taught many courses on "economic botany" at the University of California–Los Angeles and writes at length about botanical approaches to disease, leprosy probably first appeared over two millennia ago in the Nile Valley. Soldiers returning from the Crusades are believed to have been responsible for a leprosy epidemic in Europe from A.D. 1000 to 1200. Great Britain saw waves of leprosy from 625 to 1798 and at one time had 326 lazar houses—leprosariums, or hospitals for leprosy patients—within its borders. (*Lazar* is a Middle English word for leper.)

According to Professor Gibson, up until the middle of the twentieth century the only medicinal treatment for leprosy was chaulmoogra oil, which was extracted from the seeds of several trees of the family Flacourtiaceae. Chaulmoogra was first referenced as a cure for leprosy two thousand years ago, in the Hindu texts known as the Vedas. In the 1920s a botanist named Joseph Rock went to the jungles of eastern Asia for the purpose of finding trees that would yield chaulmoogra. He eventually found some in Burma, where he remained collecting plants and other specimens until, by Professor Gibson's account, he was evicted by the Chinese communists. The seeds Rock collected were sent to Hawaii and elsewhere.

Used internally and externally, chaulmoogra oil was actually successful in treating less advanced cases of leprosy and could even halt the progress of more advanced cases. Trees yielding chaulmoogra oil can still be found on the grounds of many leprosy hospitals, a reminder of bygone times. In the 1940s a drug called dapsone, taken orally, was developed and administered to thousands of leprosy patients. Today there are a number of effective remedies for the treatment of this ancient affliction.

Dumb and Furious

According to a report by the Centers for Disease Control (CDC), something mysterious happened to a twenty-nine-year-old prisoner in December of 1988.

The prisoner was working on a roadside cleanup crew in Virginia when he began experiencing back pain and malaise. The next day, complaining of abdominal cramps, vomiting, and muscle pain, he went to see the prison doctors. The doctors gave him acetaminophen, but over the next few days the prisoner's symptoms grew increasingly severe. He developed pain and tremors in his right arm, had a hard time walking, and was admitted to the hospital with a temperature of 103 degrees.

At the hospital he became agitated and began to hallucinate. He suffered from excessive salivation (foaming at the mouth) and priapism (a prolonged erection). His temperature and blood pressure fluctuated wildly. The doctors had tested him for possible pesticide poisoning from his roadside work, but the tests had come back negative. The man died several weeks later.

Another CDC report described a similar mysterious incident. Two years later, in Quebec, a nine-year-old boy woke up with a fever and a pain in his left arm. The pain did not go away, and over the next five days he developed tremors in his left arm as well as insomnia.

The boy was taken to the hospital. The doctors had no idea what was wrong with him. By the following day, the boy's condition had worsened. The tremors had spread to both arms; he began experiencing hallucinations, hydrophobia (fear of water), and other symptoms. His condition continued to deteriorate as the tremors spread, and he started to salivate excessively. He was also terribly agitated and anxious and said that he was suffocating. He died a week later.

According to the CDC, both the boy and the prisoner had been victims of rabies. Rabies is primarily a disease of the animal kingdom, but it can be transmitted to humans by an animal bite or if an infected animal's saliva touches an open wound, the mouth, or the eyes. There are only a small number of fatal cases of human rabies each year in the United States, but an estimated 40,000 people worldwide die from rabies infections each year.

In the United States, most cases of human rabies are due to bites from bats (which was suspected in the boy's case above), but other animals that can pass on rabies include dogs, cats, raccoons, skunks, coyotes, foxes, and bobcats. Most pets do not get rabies because of widespread vaccination. There has never been a documented case of rabies passed from one human to another.

Rabies is a particularly nasty way to die. Especially nasty is the fact that once rabies symptoms manifest, there is no cure, and death is, unfortunately, inevitable. A person who thinks he or she may have been bitten by a bat or other potentially infected animal needs to seek medical attention immediately, before symptoms appear. Warning signs include flulike symptoms, then paralysis of throat and face muscles and limbs, hallucinations, and extreme thirst followed by hydrophobia, and an inability to drink water. The rabies virus is said to make its victim "furious"—that is, the virus is so hungry for fresh nerve cells that it drives its victim crazy in order to make it attack, bite, and infect the next victim. Dogs can suffer from two forms of rabies: "furious" rabies and "dumb" rabies, in which paralysis renders the dog relatively immobile. Wild animals suffer from furious rabies, too, but they tend to exhibit different symptoms early on. One typical symptom is uncharacteristic behavior: For example, nocturnal animals such as bats and raccoons becoming active in daylight. The only conclusive way to test for rabies in an animal is to kill it and examine its brain.

The wolf was a common carrier of rabies in the Middle Ages. Some contemporary experts believe that many documented accounts of "mysterious wolf behavior" in those times, such as wolves attacking humans, could be attributed to rabies. Such behaviors may also be at the base of some werewolf legends (a subject that will be explored later in this book). Today, rabies is extremely rare in North American and European wolves.

One obscure but enlightening source, the Illinois Raptor Center's rabies brochure, contains an interesting historical anecdote about rabies. In medieval Europe, long before a vaccination was discovered, rabies was so feared that peasants turned to Saint Hubert, the patron saint of hunters, who is invoked against dog bites and rabies victims. Throngs of believers made pilgrimages to Liège, Belgium, to see Saint Hubert and to pray to be spared from the disease. They also used iron bars or crosses called "the keys of Saint Hubert" for additional protection against rabies. They would insert them into the walls of their houses or carry them around. If bitten by a rabid animal, many peasants would heat the keys and apply them to their wounds. If applied immediately, the wounds would often be sterilized, killing the rabies virus, which many interpreted as a miracle and further proof of Saint Hubert's divine powers. This belief in the miraculous power of the keys was held by many until well into the nineteenth century.

Another remedy believed to be effective against rabies was the root of the dog rose. In fact, this variety of wild rose was so named because it was thought to cure this disease that was so prevalent in dogs.

The nineteenth-century scientist Louis Pasteur, who invented the process of pasteurization, also discovered the rabies vaccine. In fact, Pasteur was so committed to developing a vaccine for this dreadful disease that he would often get within inches of the snapping jaws of a rabid dog in order to procure a sample of its saliva for testing and culturing.

HORRIFYING SYMPTOMS

When it comes to disease and death, none of it is pretty. But the following four medical conditions—some fatal, some not—all share the dubious distinction of having particularly awful, very unusual symptoms. Read on. . . .

TOO HOT TO HANDLE

In his book *Viruses, Plagues, and History,* Professor Michael B.
A. Oldstone relayed a mysterious and deadly chain of events
that was first reported in the May 22, 1995, issue of *Newsweek*
magazine.

In April of 1995, a thirty-six-year-old lab technician
checked into the hospital in Kikwit, a town of half a million
people in southern Zaire (now the Democratic Republic of
the Congo). The lab technician said he was suffering from
diarrhea and a fever. Doctors initially assumed that he had
dysentery, which was common in the city at that time. But
when the lab technician began bleeding from every orifice in
his body—his ears, his mouth, and his anus—the doctors realized that they had something far more severe than dysentery
on their hands. Despite their efforts to save him, he died
within four days. The mysterious sickness had turned all his
internal organs into liquid.

A nurse and a nun who had taken care of the poor man also
became sick. The nun was transferred seventy miles to another
town, where she passed the disease to several other nuns before
she died. Back in the city of Kikwit, the disease spread like
wildfire through the hospital. Terrified residents fled the city,
only to carry the illness to nearby towns and villages.

The World Health Organization was asked to respond to
this medical emergency. A team of virus hunters was sent to
Kikwit, bearing bubble suits and high-tech lab equipment. By
the time they arrived at the Kikwit hospital, it was totally

abandoned—except for a few people who had contracted the disease and were too sick to leave.

In the meantime the army had blocked the roads to prevent anyone else from leaving Kikwit. Still, despite these efforts at stopping the spread of disease, it began to move ominously toward the capital city of Kinshasa. (About 4 million of the country's 45 million people lived there.) Fortunately, the epidemic burned out before it raged completely out of control. However, it took several hundred lives before it was through, and probably more, since no one could count the number of infected people who may have died in the bush.

The virus responsible for this tragedy was a question-marked organism dubbed the Ebola virus, after the nearby Ebola River. Scientists had not seen it since 1976, when it killed several hundred people in northern Zaire. Ebola is one of a nasty group of diseases called the viral hemorrhagic fevers that includes hantavirus fever, Marburg fever, and Lassa fever. These fevers are known for their gruesome symptoms, such as uncontrollable bleeding from every opening in the body, severe diarrhea, and vomiting. Compared to the others, Ebola and Marburg are the worst germs in the bunch. The Marburg virus was so named because of an unfortunate incident in Marburg, Germany, in 1967, in which seven people died of a mysterious illness. All the cases were traced to exposure to infected African green monkeys that had been shipped from Uganda.

In comparison, hantavirus infections can sometimes be very mild and Lassa fever may not even produce noticeable symptoms. Still, there have been severe cases of both Lassa and hantavirus. Professor Oldstone's book describes vivid examples of both.

His Lassa virus anecdote, drawn originally from a report that appeared in a medical journal in the 1970s, goes back to 1969. One day, a nurse named Ms. Wine who was working in a small mission hospital in Lassa, Nigeria, complained of a backache and sore throat. A week later the doctors found several small ulcers in her throat and mouth and she was bleeding from her orifices. Eventually her speech became slurred, and she was increasingly drowsy. She was transferred to a larger hospital, Bingham Memorial Hospital, in Jos, Nigeria.

A staff nurse at Bingham Memorial, Ms. Shaw, had a small cut on her finger from picking roses for a patient. Unaware of the cut, she tended to Ms. Wine, who had just been admitted, and used the finger to hold a gauze dressing with which she swabbed the inside of Ms. Wine's mouth. When Ms. Shaw realized later that she had a small cut on that finger, she washed it and applied antiseptic to it.

The next day the patient Ms. Wine was dead. Eight days later Ms. Shaw came down with a sore throat, headache, and back and leg pains. Her symptoms continued to worsen: chills, fever, nausea, a rash, and blood oozing from various places on her body. She died within a few days.

A third nurse, Ms. Pinneo, who had tended to both nurses, came down with the symptoms as well. By this point the local doctors and health officials were alarmed that some mysterious epidemic was gaining a foothold. And so Ms. Pinneo was sent across the ocean, under extreme precautions, to New York City's Columbia University Presbyterian Hospital for medical care.

Ms. Pinneo eventually recovered. However, Dr. Cassals, who was working with specimens from Ms. Pinneo's body at the Yale University Arbovirus Research Laboratory, came down with symptoms similar to hers and the other two nurses'. On the theory that Ms. Pinneo's blood would contain anti-bodies against the virus, he was given an injection of it. The treatment worked, and Dr. Cassals survived. In fact, he contin-ued working with and studying the live Lassa fever virus, as it was now dubbed, in his laboratory.

Unfortunately, a lab technician who worked near Dr. Cas-sals's laboratory came down with Lassa fever symptoms several months later, while out of town. He died in a local hospital before he could receive the blood-antibody treatment Dr. Cas-sals had received.

The live Lassa fever virus study was discontinued at Yale. The virus was considered by many as being "too hot to handle."

Hantavirus fever can likewise come and go in small but deadly outbreaks. Professor Oldstone's book describes a fairly recent example. In 1993 two residents of the Navajo reservation in Canyon del Muerto, Arizona, became sick. The man and the woman, both young and in good health, came down suddenly with similar symptoms: cough, headache, aching muscles, and high fever. The woman's lungs soon filled with fluid, and she died of respiratory failure. The man died five days after that.

Health officials discovered that there were twenty similar cases of acute respiratory distress in the Four Corners area of the United States, where the states of New Mexico, Arizona, Utah, and Colorado meet, all twenty cases involving healthy young adults. Half of them died, and the diagnosis was han-tavirus fever.

As scary as these illnesses are, it's important not to panic or succumb to sensationalistic rumors. For example: According to the "Health-Related Hoaxes and Rumors" link on the Centers for Disease Control and Prevention's Web site (www.cdc. gov/hoax_rumors.htm), an e-mail was being circulated suggesting that hantavirus could be spread via canned foods or packaged foods. The e-mail specifically mentioned a U.S. stock clerk who became infected with hantavirus while working in a stockroom; the e-mail went on to caution readers about handling items such as soda cans or packaged foods such as cereal boxes because they may be contaminated with hantavirus-filled rodent droppings or the like. The case mentioned in the e-mail has never been verified by the CDC.

MAD HUMAN DISEASE

Robert M. Youngson's book *Medical Curiosities* contains a particularly gruesome story about bulking up gone wrong.

A buff young professional bodybuilder was eager to get even buffer, and his regular workouts weren't doing it for him anymore. So he decided to kick it up a notch by giving himself a series of injections of human growth hormone, derived from the pituitary gland, which he had heard could be even more powerful than anabolic steroids in enhancing muscle development. After asking around, he found a Hungarian source for the hormone.

After a period of using the hormone, the young bodybuilder began developing mysterious symptoms: severe headaches, joint pains, and difficulty walking, talking, and swallowing. Eventually he was hospitalized and diagnosed with Creutzfeldt-Jakob disease. He died three weeks later. A medical expert testified that there had been cases of people contracting this disease as a result of using growth hormone derived from cadavers.

Creutzfeldt-Jakob disease (CJD) is a rare, degenerative brain disorder characterized by rapidly progressive neurological and neuromuscular symptoms. Symptoms include confusion, depression, loss of motor control, shocklike muscle spasms, slow writhing movements (particularly of the arms and legs), dementia, susceptibility to pneumonia and other upper-respiratory infections, paralysis, and eventually death.

CJD and a number of other degenerative brain diseases are believed to be caused by protein particles that lack nucleic acid and are thought to be infectious agents. CJD is one of the many so-called prion diseases, often referred to as spongiform encephalopathies, which all share the characteristic of eating away at mammalian brains. This group includes scrapie, which affects sheep; transmissible mink encephalopathy; chronic wasting disease of mule deer and elk; bovine spongiform encephalopathy (BSE), or mad cow disease; and Gerstmann-Straussler-Scheinker disease, fatal familial insomnia, kuru, and Alpers syndrome, all of which affect humans.

In most cases, CJD appears to occur for no particular reason. In some cases there is a hereditary component. In rare instances, CJD is thought to be an infectious disease in which prions invade the brain. Some cases have been traced to treatments via products that come from human tissue, such as human growth hormone injections, as in the case of the bodybuilder.

In the 1990s, a variant form of CJD called V–CJD, V standing for *variant*, surfaced in the United Kingdom. Some experts suggest that V–CJD is linked to mad cow disease, and may be caused by human consumption of BSE-tainted beef. CJD is sometimes referred to as the human version of mad cow disease.

Diagnosis of CJD is very difficult and can only be achieved by means of a brain biopsy—or an autopsy, at which point it is too late. Furthermore, a diagnosis is not particularly useful, as there is no cure for CJD, and approximately 90 percent of CJD patients die within a first year of diagnosis. Treatment consists of trying to make the patient as comfortable as possible and to alleviate the symptoms. CJD tends to affect people over the age of fifty. However, V–CJD affects a younger population; the median age tends to be around the late twenties.

Mad cow disease and all its nasty relatives have led to international panic, slaughter of thousands of animals, boycotts on beef, concerns about the human blood supply, and more. Fortunately, cases of CJD continue to be extremely few and far between, although the unfortunate one in a million who contracts it will suffer terribly.

THE FLESH-EATING BUG

At first, it appears to be the flu. You have a high fever, sore throat, chills, nausea, and a general ill feeling. At the same time you may notice that some spot on your body is a bit sore. There may be a cut or scratch there. You don't take much notice of it.

A day or two later, your "flu" gets worse. The soreness on that spot has progressed to "serious pain." The spot eventually starts to swell; a purplish rash may appear, as well as big, dark blisters filled with blackish fluid.

Days later the pain is excruciating. The swelling is atrocious, and the skin over the spot may have split open. Cloudy liquid that looks like dishwater oozes out. You may or may not float in and out of consciousness.

The pain then changes to total numbness, since your nerves are now kaput—gone. You become delirious; you cannot urinate at all; you can barely breathe. Your organs go into toxic shock and shut down. Your skin and other tissues turn black and fall off your body.

This terrible condition, dubbed "the flesh-eating bug" by the popular media, is necrotizing fasciitis. According to the book *Surviving the "Flesh-Eating Bacteria"* by Jacqueline A. Roemmele and Donna Batdorff, necrotizing fasciitis, which means "decaying flesh," is most commonly caused by the same bacterium that causes strep throat. It can enter the body through a scratch, paper cut, pinprick, bruise, blister, or other minor skin injury.

Necrotizing fasciitis can be fatal. Survivors may face partial skin removal or even amputation of fingers and toes, limbs, and, in some cases, breasts and genitals (males).

BLOWFISH POISONING

In Japan, eating blowfish—also referred to as puffer fish—could be considered the height of culinary sophistication or the height of macho stupidity, depending on how you look at it. Called *fugu* in Japanese, the blowfish is one of the most poisonous fish in the world. Unless the fish is prepared by a specially licensed *fugu* chef who knows exactly what he or she is doing and removes the toxic parts properly—liver, gonads, intestines, and skin—the *fugu* eater will surely die a quick and terrible death involving respiratory paralysis, convulsions, and more.

The deadly parts of the fish contain tetrodotoxin, a powerful neurotoxin. Just to put things in context, tetrodotoxin is 150,000 times more deadly than strychnine. Some claim that tetrodotoxin is one of the ingredients in the voodoo potion used in zombie rituals.

By some accounts, three thousand Japanese citizens suffered from *fugu* poisoning from 1955 to 1975, and half of these died. Approximately fifty Japanese still perish from *fugu* poisoning each year. Yet people continue to play culinary Russian roulette and order it at restaurants. It is apparently a great culinary delicacy. There is a saying: "Those who eat *fugu* soup are stupid; those who do not eat *fugu* soup are also stupid."

Indeed, the Japanese cannot seem to get enough of the stuff. According to an entertaining Web site article entitled "*Fugu*: The Deadly Delicacy" (by a writer named simply Musashi), one market in the Japanese town of Shimonoseki reportedly makes $40 million every winter just from *fugu* sales. Incidentally, *fugu* is sold live, unlike other fish that are packed dead or nearly dead on ice. Because the creatures are so ferocious and aggressive, the fishermen must sew their mouths shut in order to keep them from killing each other.

Matsuo Bashō, a seventeenth-century Japanese poet, eloquently described the existential joy he felt after eating blowfish one evening—and living to see daylight:

So! Nothing at all happened!
Yesterday has vanished
After blowfish soup.

BIG, BIGGER, BIGGEST

Robert Pershing Wadlow, dubbed "the Gentle Giant" and "the Alton Giant," was eight feet eleven inches and 490 pounds at the time of his death. According to the Web site of the Alton Museum of History and Art in Alton, Illinois, where Wadlow grew up, Wadlow was five feet six and a half inches at age five, when he entered kindergarten, and he wore the clothes of a boy age seventeen. By age eight he was six feet two inches and weighed 185 pounds. He continued his bizarre growth spurts until he died in 1940 at age twenty-two.

Another famous "giant" was Andre Roussimoff, known in World Wrestling Federation circles as Andre the Giant. Born in Grenoble, France, in 1946, Andre was six feet three inches at the age of twelve; in adulthood he towered at seven feet, five inches and weighed more than 500 pounds. According to the Manly-web Web site, Andre the Giant beat Hulk Hogan on a number of occasions. He died in 1993 at the age of forty-six. The same year the WWF inducted him into their wrestling Hall of Fame.

Both Robert Pershing Wadlow and Andre the Giant suffered from a childhood disease known as gigantism. Gigantism is characterized by exaggerated bone growth and excessive height, and is caused by excess production of growth hormone.

Acromegaly is a close relative of gigantism that affects adults. It is a rare condition in which certain bones in the body grow much bigger than they should. It, too, is caused by over-production of growth hormone by the pituitary gland and may result from a pituitary tumor. Bones in the face, hands, feet, and elsewhere, as well as the tongue and other soft tissues, can become noticeably enlarged. These changes happen very slowly over time, often making diagnosis difficult.

Treatment for acromegaly can range from drugs to radiation therapy and surgery, if there is a pituitary tumor involved. However, though soft tissues such as the tongue may gradually decrease in size with treatment, the enlarged bones will never go back to the way they were.

UNCOMMON NAMES FOR UNCOMMON DISEASES

The next nine disorders have the dubious distinction of having very unusual names. They are fortunately extremely rare, because in addition to being unpleasant illnesses with unpleasant symptoms, they do not exactly trip off the tongue. Unless otherwise noted, they were mostly culled from the fascinating Web site of the National Organization for Rare Disorders (www.rarediseases.org).

CAT-EYE SYNDROME

Cat-eye syndrome is a rare chromosomal disorder that can result in widely spaced eyes, eyelid folds that slant downward, and other eye defects. Other possible symptoms include malformed ears and, mysteriously, the absence of a normal anal canal. This latter symptom causes the large intestine to connect up with the bladder, vagina, or other inappropriate organ instead of the anus. Some victims of this disease suffer from only mild symptoms; others suffer from a wide range of severe ones.

VIBRATION WHITE FINGER

This disorder sounds kind of naughty, but it's not what you think. According to the *American College of Physicians Complete Home Medical Guide*, vibration white finger, also known as hand-arm syndrome, is a condition caused by excessive exposure to vibrating machinery. Symptoms include pale or blue fingers, difficulty in handling small objects or performing other small motor-control activities such as tying shoelaces or buttoning clothes, and pain, numbness, and tingling in the afflicted limbs.

In the past, workers in the mining and engineering industries represented a majority of vibration white finger cases. Today, people who operate chainsaws on a day-to-day basis—say, workers in the forestry industry or Leatherface from *The Texas Chainsaw Massacre*—tend to be the primary victims.

CHRISTMAS DISEASE

No, this illness is not caused by maxing out all your credit cards, drinking too much eggnog, or having to spend the long holiday weekend in Detroit with your in-laws. A condition that affects only males, Christmas disease, named for the first man who was diagnosed, is a close but far rarer cousin of hemophilia. According to the *American College of Physicians Complete Home Medical Guide*, Christmas disease is caused by the deficiency of a protein that is involved in the clotting of blood.

As with hemophilia, symptoms of Christmas disease include prolonged bleeding, say, bleeding from a small cut for hours or even days, blood in the urine, and sudden swelling of joints and muscles as a result of internal bleeding. Christmas disease is treatable to some extent, depending on the severity of the condition; bleeding problems can be managed with clotting-factor replacement therapy, which is done by injection.

KABUKI MAKEUP SYNDROME (KMS)

This disorder, also called Kabuki syndrome or Niikawaku-roki syndrome, is a rare disorder characterized by a range of peculiar symptoms including skeletal abnormalities, short stature, and mental retardation. Also, one's facial features grow distorted, and the fingers, toes, the palms of the hands, and the soles of the feet become covered with strange skin-ridge patterns. The syndrome was named by the Japanese doctors who first diagnosed it because the facial symptoms resembled the makeup of actors of the traditional Japanese theater known as Kabuki. The cause of this syndrome is unknown at this time.

JUMPING FRENCHMEN OF MAINE

This disorder, also referred to as jumping Frenchmen, *latah* in Malaysia, and *myriachit* in Siberia, is characterized by an extreme startle reaction to an unexpected noise, sight, or other stimulus. Patients—more often males than females—will jump, flail their arms, hit something or someone, cry out, or repeat words. The startle reaction can be exacerbated by fatigue or stress.

It was first identified in Maine and in the Canadian province of Quebec in the nineteenth century when it was observed in Maine lumberjacks of French-Canadian origin. No one has pinpointed why those lumberjacks were susceptible to this disorder, and subsequently, jumping Frenchmen of Maine has been observed in other groups in different parts of the world. It may be a hereditary neurological disorder, although cultural or social influence may play a part as well.

Maple Syrup Urine Disease

This illness is *not* caused by eating too many buckwheat pancakes. It is, instead, a very rare inherited metabolic disorder in which one's urine and sweat have a very sweet odor caused by the body's inability to break down, or metabolize, the amino acids leucine, isoleucine, and valine, which are essential for building proteins and other purposes.

Lest you think Maple Syrup Urine disease is silly-sounding, you should know that it can be fatal if not treated quickly and appropriately. You might also try calling it by one of its other, more serious names: branched-chain ketoaciduria.

Prune–Belly Syndrome

"Prune belly" is not just a mean nickname for your overweight spouse. It is a rare disease of unknown cause and is characterized by the complete or partial absence of the abdominal muscles, bilateral cryptorchidism (undescended testicles), and a malformed urinary tract. Prune belly syndrome is also referred to as abdominal muscle deficiency syndrome, congenital absence of the abdominal muscles, Eagle-Barrett syndrome, and Obrinsky syndrome. It is a congenital disease whose incidence is approximately 1 in 40,000 live births. It can cause terrible complications with urinary, renal, respiratory, and other bodily functions.

Prune-belly syndrome is so named because it gives the abdomen a wrinkly, puckered appearance. It can also give the appearance of a severe pot belly, one that not only extends out but droops down toward the ground.

HAIRY TONGUE

According to the *American College of Physicians Complete Home Medical Guide,* unfortunate victims of hairy tongue—sometimes referred to as black hairy tongue, black tongue, *lingua nigra,* and *lingua villosa nigra*—suffer from a tongue that is discolored and whose filiform papillae grow abnormally long. It is an uncommon and fairly benign condition (except for the possible negative nose-dive effect on one's love life).

The cause is not known at this time, although several theories have been posed, including poor oral hygiene, smoking, chewing tobacco, and the like.

WANDERING SPLEEN

Wandering spleen is an extremely rare birth defect in which the ligaments holding the spleen in its normal position are underdeveloped or missing altogether. This leads the spleen to wander in the lower abdomen and pelvic area and wreak some serious havoc, causing abdominal pain, vomiting, nausea, fatigue, and more.

Also known as displaced spleen, drifting spleen, floating spleen, and a number of other colorful names, wandering spleen can also be acquired in adulthood as a result of illness, injury, or a condition such as pregnancy (as if not being able to fit into one's clothes and having to pee ten times in the middle of the night weren't enough).

FREAKS OF NATURE

People have always been fascinated and disgusted by so-called freaks of nature who possess too many body parts, not enough body parts, strange growths sprouting out of their heads, and so forth. In a 1937 book entitled *Anomalies and Curiosities of Medicine: An Encyclopedic Collection of Rare and Extraordinary Cases and of the Most Striking Instances of Abnormality in All Branches of Medicine and Surgery, Derived from an Exhaustive Research of Medical Literature from Its Origin to the Present Day, Abstracted, Classified, Annotated, and Indexed*, George M. Gould and Walter L. Pyle discuss hundreds of cases of genuine freakishness. Their book includes the following entries:

- A 20-year-old woman who menstruated from her breast, and other cases of women who menstruated from their ears, eyes, and mouths
- An 18-year-old woman who had been menstruating since age 3

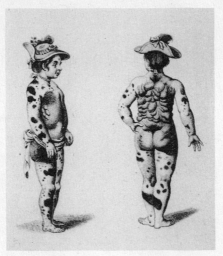

- Menstruating men
- A woman who carried a (dead) fetus in her uterus for forty-six years
- Three-headed men
- Men with two penises
- Men with horns growing out of their heads
- The Four-Eyed Man of Cricklade, who had two pairs of eyes
- A woman with ten breasts
- Men and women with ears growing out of their necks and chests
- Women who had worms, maggots, and snakes in their uteruses
- Pregnant women with strange food cravings: for plaster, charcoal, cloth, excrement, human flesh, and human blood

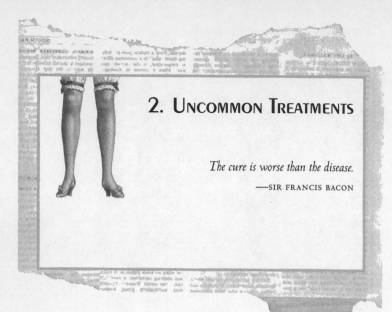

2. Uncommon Treatments

The cure is worse than the disease.

—SIR FRANCIS BACON

As long as there have been diseases, there have been attempts at treatment, successful and unsuccessful. Throughout the ages and in all the cultures of the world, healers and laypersons have grappled with their understanding of the human body and disease, often stretching the concept of medicine to include experimentation with poisonous plants, animal extracts, mysterious chants, gems and minerals, bodily waste, and more. In both scientific and folk-medicine experiments, most of these efforts were driven by a genuine desire to heal; others were driven by a desire for profit, as "snake-oil salesmen" and their equivalents sought to make a quick buck from the sick and desperate.

This chapter presents a sampling of some of the most uncommon treatments, cures, and remedies from different points in history. Many of these treatments have been passed down through the generations, even as medical science has either proved or disproved their effectiveness. Some of the most bizarre and harmful treatments have, thankfully, been abandoned as more effective remedies have been discovered. And among the remedies that are still prevalent today are what were once radical or experimental treatments that have become confirmed medical convention; still others continue to exist on the fringe of medical convention with nothing but anecdotal evidence of their usefulness.

FIRST, DO NO HARM

Born around 460 B.C. in Greece, Hippocrates is widely considered to be the father of medicine. However, very little is known about his life, or even about his exact identity; in fact, there may have been more than one man by that name. Alternatively, Hippocrates may have authored none, or only some, of the writings that make up the *Corpus Hippocraticum,* or Hippocratic Collection.

Whatever the case, the writings credited to Hippocrates not only elevated the science of medicine during his time but continued to be important and valid for thousands of years. In those writings, it was first established that the role of the physician was to "first, do no harm." By observing sick people, Hippocrates was able to note and record symptoms of grave illness, ascertain the importance of listening to the breath through the chest, and more. He may have been the first advocate of the second opinion. And, of course, his rules for the conduct of doctors—known as the Hippocratic oath—are still muttered by medical students at graduation ceremonies everywhere.

Not all medical innovators are as well remembered as Hippocrates, however, or as well regarded. And many of the treatments doctors and other healers prescribed were not only ineffective but did far more damage than the sickness itself.

BLOODLETTING

Although Hippocrates is credited with transforming the practice of medicine into a science, many of his treatments were based on the doctrine of the four humors: blood, phlegm, black bile, and yellow bile. In order for a person to be well, it was necessary for these four humors to be balanced. As the theory developed over time—beginning with the ancient Greeks and remaining popular throughout the Middle Ages— the humors were often compared with, or somehow connected to, the four seasons; the quadrants of the zodiac (four groups of three signs); the compass directions north, south, east, and west; the four evangelists John, Luke, Matthew, and Mark; the four stages of life (infancy, adolescence, adulthood, and old age); and more. Most foods, plants, and even household items were specified as being dry, wet, hot, or cold so they could be applied to the body in such a way as to balance the humors appropriately.

The importance of the blood being in balance with the rest of the body led to the practice of bleeding patients as a common form of treatment for a vast number of ailments. According to the theory, each organ was believed to correspond with certain veins; opening these veins was thought to draw toxic humors away from the unwell organs. There were different methods of drawing blood: derivation, or letting the blood out close to the affected place, and revulsion, or letting the blood out very far from the affected place. Many different tools were employed in bloodletting: A patient was bled either through the use of leeches or through a lancet or other blade to pierce the skin. Unfortunately, bloodletting led to more damage and death than healing, as a result of accidental cutting of nerves and arteries, not to mention loss of blood.

Bloodletting had strong scientific backing while it was practiced. Aulus Cornelius Celsus, a renowned Roman medical writer, was one of the first major advocates of bloodletting. Around the first-century A.D., Celsus crafted *De medicina*, a medical treatise containing important information on the surgery of that era, anatomy, the repair of fractures, the restoration of the foreskin after circumcision, catheterization, and of course bloodletting. According to Robert M. Youngson's book *Medical Curiosities*, much of *De medicina* may have been borrowed liberally from the writings of Hippocrates and another

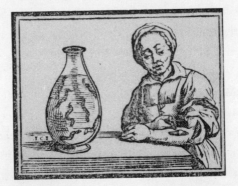

physician. But Hippocrates himself was not a big fan of bloodletting, while Celsus believed in using it to treat everything but the kitchen sink, including breathlessness, redness of the skin, convulsions, and chronic weakness. So even though Celsus may have made significant contributions to medicine, his passionate advocacy of bloodletting was not one of them, and may have led to many unnecessary deaths-by-bleeding through the centuries.

MEDIEVAL MEDICINE

In the early Middle Ages, medical practices were primarily based on ancient Greek and Roman texts. Unfortunately, a lot of the lessons in these tomes were passed on to subsequent generations via less-than-accurate translations and were based on unreliable theory. During this era, medical reference books, called leechbooks, were written that described a number of illnesses and their remedies based both on ancient Greek practices and popular treatments developed at the time.

Here is a sampling of these folk remedies, taken from the Mostly Medieval Web site (www.skell.org) and an article entitled "Folk Remedies, Cures, Potions, and Charms" from the Historic-UK Web site (www.historic-uk.com). Some of them have existed since the Middle Ages; some are later evolutions of medieval remedies.

Most of these remedies are obsolete and sound outlandish to contemporary readers, but some are actually still employed today. For example, alternative healers use the herb tansy for a variety of purposes. It can be taken internally to expel intestinal parasites and flatulence, be taken as a tea to reduce fever, and used externally to relieve skin eruptions and swelling from sprains. And today, Saint-John's-wort is a popular herbal remedy for anxiety and depression.

Another popular remedy recommended by the leechbooks was oxymel, which was a type of medicinal drink that combined vinegar with honey or sugar syrup. Oxymel goes back to Hippocrates, who prescribed it a great deal to his own patients for "freedom of breathing" and other benefits. Healers in the Middle Ages recommended it for everything from jaundice and epilepsy to being "tired from a long journey" and eating bad melons. Some herbalists today still tout its effectiveness for healing and use it as an expectorant, although evidence of its benefits are vague at best. See the table on pages 59–65 on herbal remedies and their uses in the past and present.

SOME FOLK REMEDIES FROM HISTORY

Ailment	Treatment
CANCER	Make an ointment of goat's gall and honey or spread the ashes from a dog's skull over a patient's skin.
STROKE	Inhale the smoke of a burning pine tree.
GOITER AND TUMORS	Touch a hanged man's hand.
COLIC AND GALLSTONES	Wear copper rings or bracelets.
WARTS	Rub the wart with a piece of meat, then bury the meat.
BALDNESS	Sleep on stones or rub goose dung over the bald spot.
EYE PROBLEMS	Bathe the eyes with rainwater collected in June, before sunrise. Or make an eye ointment with scrapings from a fourteenth-century tomb.
STIES	Rub the sty with a gold wedding ring.

AILMENT	TREATMENT
BACTERIAL INFECTIONS	Apply a mixture of homemade wine, ox gall, garlic, and leeks that has been allowed to sit in a brass pot for nine days.
TOOTHACHES	Drive a nail into the tooth, then extract the bloody nail and pound it into a tree. The tree will then "take on" the pain. To prevent toothache, wear a dead mole around the neck.
AGUE (A FORM OF MALARIA)	Wrap a spider in a raisin and swallow. Or wear shoes lined with tansy leaves.
PAINFUL THIGHS	Apply pounded hemlock and henbane to the thighs.
PARALYSIS	Let blood and induce vomiting.
STOMACH DISEASE	Chew on laurel leaves, swallow their juice, and place the chewed-up leaves on the belly.
HEADACHE	Boil heather and apply to the top of the head while still warm.
INSOMNIA	Eat egg white and nettles mixed together.

(cont.)

AILMENT	TREATMENT
FEVER	Ingest Saint-John's-wort, especially if the plant is found by accident on midsummer's eve.
TO CURE A SICK CHILD	When the moon is waxing, cut woodbine and make it into hoops, then preserve until March. The sick child should pass through the hoop three times.
TO WARD OFF EVIL	Make a bracelet with senna, mint, and rue. Or make a wreath with convolvulus and primrose picked on the first of May.
INSANITY	Wear buttercup in a bag around the neck.
CATARACTS	Draw fresh well water and let the basin rest on wood, never on stone or earth. Add a silver or gold coin to the water, then add blades of grass. After steeping, rub the grass across the affected eye, then pour the water into the eye.
FRECKLES	Cover the freckles with blood from a bull or hare, or water distilled from crushed-up walnuts.
CRAMPS	Wrap the skin of an eel around the knees.

BARBER—SURGEONS

In the Middle Ages, before medicine became a regulated, scientific study, barbers used their dexterity with blades to provide much more than clean shaves. Many rural areas lacked trained physicians (due in part to their demise during the plague), giving way for "barber-surgeons" to perform many common medical duties such as pulling teeth, bloodletting, removing hernias, performing tonsillectomies, cesarean sections, and sometimes amputations.

Bloodletting was so widely practiced by barbers that they began advertising their specialized service with a red and white pole, signifying blood and the tourniquet, in their storefronts. Often patients actually squeezed a pole or stick to aid the flow of blood. And in colonial America, before anesthesia, fast-cutting barbers often performed lithotomies, the removal of kidney or bladder stones. These barber-surgeons, called

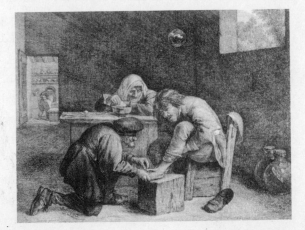

"stonecutters," would slice patients open quickly and remove the offending stones. One stonecutter gained acclaim for being able to perform a lithotomy in less than thirty seconds.

According to Gilbert R. Seigworth's article "Bloodletting over the Centuries," barbers and surgeons actually shared a trade guild in England until the mid–eighteenth century. But eventually and inevitably surgery became the sole domain of surgeons, and barbers, thank goodness, returned to the practice of cutting hair rather than veins.

MEDIEVAL MEDICAL PRACTITIONERS

Throughout the Middle Ages, many people filled different roles in the medical community on both a professional and amateur level. University-trained doctors were not available in most rural areas throughout the Middle Ages, and alternative cures were often employed, such as charms, rituals, and prayer. Many patients also had to seek out other kinds of practitioners besides barbers. Here are some examples of such practitioners, from the Mostly Medieval Web site (www.skell.org):

- **Monks and priests.** Monks copied manuscripts of the writings of Hippocrates and other ancient medical experts. In the early Middle Ages, they were thought to have practiced what they scribed; some became such skilled healers that patients sought out their services in addition to, or instead of, the services of physicians. At that time all monasteries had infirmaries to treat the sick, the elderly, and the indigent, as well as travelers passing through. But in the early thirteenth century, the Catholic Church ruled that priests could no longer shed blood, making way for barbers, already skilled with blades, and other laypersons to take on the responsibility of bloodletting and other minor surgery.

- **Leeches.** Not to be confused with the slimy little creatures used in bloodletting procedures, *leech* was also a term used for a lay healer who practiced without any sort of formal education. Leeches sometimes acted as apprentices to barber-surgeons or physicians.
- *Dentatores.* Only the rich and famous could afford the services of these medieval dentists. Their primary duties were removing decay, believed to be caused by worms, and filling teeth with ground bone from oxen and other animals, and later with gold.
- **Herbalists.** The profiles and practice of herbalists and other folk healers varied widely across Europe. In some areas the herbalists were mostly women; in others, mostly men. Likewise, in some areas, healing secrets were passed on from woman to woman only; in others, from man to man. Some people believed that an herbalist was "born" with his or her healing skills and that these skills would be rendered ineffective in the hands of someone not a natural-born healer.

ARTHRITIS "CURES"

The pursuit of effective pain relief throughout history has fostered some of the most creative remedies in folk medicine,

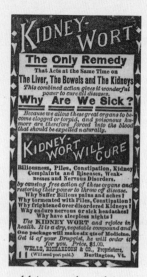

especially remedies to treat arthritis pain. Arthritis is notoriously difficult to treat, with pain that comes and goes, increases and decreases in intensity, and ultimately has no cure, even today. Throughout history, treatments for arthritis have ranged from the potentially harmful, such as extracting bad teeth (believed to be the cause of the affliction) and sitting in a uranium mine, to the harmless yet totally ineffective, such as carrying buckshot or a potato in one's pocket, rubbing snake oil into one's joints, or drinking a mixture of water and turtle ashes.

Not all old-time arthritis remedies have proved to be bogus, however. One such exception is the use of white willow bark. Historical references to the medicinal use of willow bark date from around 500 B.C., when the Chinese used the plant as a pain reliever, probably in a tea. Hippocrates advised that willow bark and leaves should be chewed to alleviate pain and fever. But it wasn't until the nineteenth century that medical technology caught up with this folk remedy and discovered that the active ingredient in willow is the chemical salicin, which is similar to salicylic acid. Salicylic acid was found to be an effective painkiller, and fifty years after this initial discovery, Bayer began marketing the purified compound of salicylic acid as aspirin for the treatment of pain and arthritis.

But even aspirin cannot relieve the pain that afflicts many arthritis sufferers. To this day an array of alternative treatments for arthritis exist, and American consumers spend a great deal of money on unproven arthritis "cures" ranging from the old standards of snake oil and wearing copper bracelets to magnet therapy and bee venom. Many people swear by the effectiveness of bee venom treatment, which involves allowing oneself to get stung by bees in order to alleviate arthritis pain. Bee venom is believed to contain peptides that have anti-inflammatory properties. People who may be allergic to bees or who don't know whether they are should (obviously) consult their physicians before undergoing this treatment.

ABOUT GOUT

Gout is a particularly painful form of arthritis. In ancient times, gouty arthritis was believed to be a "rich man's disease" because a diet heavy in pork, beer, and port was suspected to be the cause. Indeed, we now know that one factor that can exacerbate gout is a diet high in purines, chemicals that can be found in organ meats and yeast.

Many bizarre cures have been used throughout history in an attempt to alleviate the painful symptoms of gout. The ancient Greeks believed that dysentery (bloody diarrhea) may actually cure gout. In accordance with this theory, patients were exposed to a person with dysentery or themselves ingested contaminated food or water. A seventeenth-century doctor recommended wool compresses soaked in hot "frogge water," a concoction of frog eggs aged for several weeks. Until the nineteenth century, sex was believed to be one of the causes of gout, leading many gout sufferers to abstain; some doctors

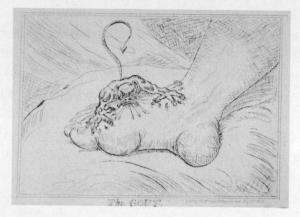

The GOUT.

even went to the lengths of prescribing castration. Perhaps the most disturbing remedy was the medieval recipe of roast goose stuffed with chopped-up kittens.

THE MAGIC OF BEZOAR

Bezoar is a sort of reddish stone, although *stone* is a misnomer. Bezoar is in actuality a rock-hard hairball or gallstone from the stomach of an animal such as a goat or llama and sometimes, a human. Derived from two Persian words meaning "against" and "poison," bezoar was believed from medieval times on to be a powerful antidote to poisoning. In order to work, bezoar had to be taken orally, rubbed over the body, or worn. So valuable were these stones at one time that they were known to fetch ten times their weight in gold.

One strange legend attributes the powers of bezoar to Oriental stags. When the stags reached a certain age, they were said to eat serpents in order to regain their youth. But in consuming the serpents, the stags consumed their venom as well. To detoxify quickly, the stags ran into a stream while keeping their heads above water. This action somehow caused fluid to be distilled from their eyes, and the fluid was then transformed into bezoar by the heat of the sun.

In his 1653 volume *Complete Herbal*, Nicholas Culpepper, an English apothecary, wrote:

> Take of Pearls prepared, Crab's eyes, red Coral, white Amber Hart's-horn, oriental Bezoar, of each half an ounce, powder of the black tops of Crab's claws, the weight of them all, beat them into powder, which may be made into balls with jelly, and the skins which our vipers have cast off, warily dried and kept for use . . . Four, or five, or six grains is excellently good in a fever to be taken in any cordial, for it cheers the heart and vital spirits exceedingly, and makes them impregnable.

Bezoar didn't always bring about happy results, however. According to Robert M. Youngson's book *Medical Curiosities*, there is a story about King Charles IX of France, who ruled in the mid–sixteenth century and was a great believer in the healing effects of bezoar. In fact, the king had a stone of which he was particularly proud. But the French barber-surgeon Ambroise Paré wished to convince the king that rock-hard hairballs and other similar substances had no healing effects whatsoever. To this end, Paré suggested an experiment to the king. A cook had been condemned to death for stealing, and Paré told the king to give the cook a choice: He could be publicly strangled, or he could take a fatal poison and then be cured by the king's bezoar stone.

The cook agreed to the latter option and was subsequently given a large dose of a corrosive poison, bichloride of mercury, immediately followed by a treatment with the bezoar stone. Within an hour the cook was in the throes of agony, and attempts were made to treat him with the stone. He reportedly suffered from vomiting, pain, bloody diarrhea, and kidney failure for seven horrific hours before dying. After the ordeal the king ordered Paré to burn the bezoar.

THE HAIR OF THE DOG

Alcohol has been used as a medicinal treatment in many ways throughout history, but never with much success. A seventeenth-century Puritan minister named Cotton Mather, renowned for his expertise in science and the supernatural, recommended a glass of wine along with a few grains of rat dung to treat diarrhea. Reverend Mather had other interesting ideas for medicinal remedies. For example, he believed in the medicinal properties of onions to relieve muscle pain; he recommended boiling them, draining them, mashing them to a pulp,

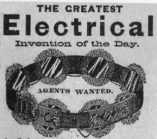

and applying them as a poultice "as hott as the Patient can bear."

   .   According to Robert M. Youngson's *Medical Curiosities,* Robert Bentley Todd, a nineteenth-century professor of physiology at King's College in London, England, believed in using alcohol for medical purposes. He believed that a number of diseases could be treated with the careful administration of alcohol—a treatment that he employed with his patients and on himself. One day he began vomiting blood, and within two days he was dead. The postmortem showed that he had advanced cirrhosis of the liver.

ARSENIC

Arsenic has a long history of medicinal uses, despite the fact that it was well known to be extremely poisonous in large doses. However, throughout much of history it was believed that careful administration of arsenic was not dangerous and in fact had many healthful benefits. In Hippocrates's time, it was used to treat malaria and syphilis. (Syphilis has a tradition of being treated with poisons: In the Middle Ages, it was also treated with mercury.) When given over a period of time in small doses, arsenic does cure venereal disease and can, in many cases, be tolerated. Until the mid–twentieth century it was the most effective known treatment, but thankfully the use of arsenic became outmoded once more effective antibiotics were developed.

Today we are still exposed to small amounts of arsenic through our environment in drinking water, hospital labs, metal alloys, taxidermy preservatives, growth promoters for livestock, and an agent that removes color from glass. Studies are still being conducted on the medicinal uses of arsenic. It has been found effective in fighting certain types of leukemia and other cancers. However, it has also been found to be a carcinogen.

FOLK REMEDIES

Folk remedies made from herbs and other healing recipes made from substances found around the home have been around for many centuries. A number of them are still used today, whether because of family or community traditions, a need for alternatives to conventional medicine, or long-standing cultural and historical practice, as in the cases of Chinese medicine and Indian Ayurvedic medicine. In the United States, Native Americans have an ancient tradition of healing practices such as sweat lodges, communal dancing, and prayer.

As in the example of willow bark, many folk remedies have withstood the test of modern medical science and have been proved effective treatments, either on their own or as complementary therapy. Other therapies have withstood the test of time as well, yet remain on the fringes of today's alternative medical practice. At a time when alternative and complementary therapies are gaining acceptance, it is difficult to ignore the champions of many of these therapies. Yet, even in

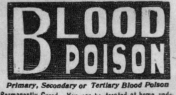

a climate of increasing acceptance of alternative therapies, many of these treatments retain their air of curiosity and have not crossed over into widespread acceptance.

The History of Medicinal Plants

Even before Hippocrates, plants were employed for medicinal purposes, and they continue to be so employed today. The history books suggest that around 3000 B.C., the Babylonians were already using myrrh medicinally. The Chinese and Indians were also using plants for medicine thousands of years ago, as were Native Americans. It's reasonable to assume that even earlier societies of hunters and gatherers experimented with plants for healing. The table "Herbs in History" (below) reveals some popular medicinal herbs from history and how their use developed over time.

HERBS IN HISTORY		
Herb	**Historical use**	**Present use**
Angelica	Stomachache, colds, cough, fever, and plague.	Fights viral and bacterial infections, reduces fever, strengthens bones.
		(cont.)

Herb	Historical use	Present use
BASIL, THYME, OR CALAMINT	The sixteenth-century herbalist John Gerard prescribed this for serpent bites, bruises, and burns.	Oil can be used in warm baths to soothe and to relieve toothaches.
BEE BALM (BERGAMOT)	A popular herb used in tea by Native Americans for treatment of colic, gas, fever, cold, stomach problems, insomnia, heart trouble, nosebleeds. Once believed to expel worms.	Used in aromatherapy for its fragrance, which is said to be calming, and for its minty flavor in teas. It is still used medicinally by some to treat fever, stomach problems, and insomnia.
BLOODROOT	Men of the Ponca tribe were known to rub bloodroot on their hands, then shake hands with the woman they wanted to marry. It was used as a dye and medicinally for fever and rheumatism, and as an emetic.	Expectorant for treatment of respiratory problems and asthma.
BLUE FLAG (IRIS)	For cleansing blood and treating migraines.	A mild expectorant for treating respiratory problems
BUTTERFLY WEED	Native Americans made the root into a paste to treat sores.	Treats digestive disorders

herb	historical use	present use
CARDINAL FLOWER (LOBELIA)	Its traditional use as an expectorant is evident in the plant's other common names: pukeweed, gagroot, and vomitwort.	Used in homeopathy to treat asthma; can be used to help break addiction to smoking.
CATNIP	Leaves were chewed to cure headaches and toothaches; brewed in tea for treating insomnia, headache, stomachache, and bronchitis.	Prevents hives, reduces fever, soothes measles and chicken pox, treats the flu and insomnia.
CELANDINE	Used to treat skin conditions such as blisters, warts, and rashes; also for jaundice and liver ailments.	Treats liver and gallbladder complaints and loss of appetite.
COMFREY	Used to treat dysentery, sprains, bruises, broken bones.	Used topically to relieve pain and inflammation and to treat bruises and sprains.
CULVER'S ROOT	A laxative.	The aged root is used as a laxative, to induce sweating, to stimulate the liver, and as a diuretic.

(cont.)

Herb	Historical use	Present use
DITTANY OF CRETE (MARJORAM)	Was used in wine to treat diseases of the head; also to treat gas, toothaches, and speed up childbirth as well as the flow of menstrual blood.	Treats sprains and bruises.
FEVERFEW	Has been used since the first century to treat headaches.	Treats headaches, inflammation, fever, and arthritis.
FOXGLOVE	Use originated in Ireland to treat ulcers, boils, headaches, paralysis, and high blood pressure.	Considered today to be poisonous.
FRINGE TREE	For inflammations, sores, cuts, and infections.	Treats liver and gall-bladder conditions, including gallstones.
GINSENG	American and Chinese ginseng have many similar properties. In America, Native Americans used this to treat nausea and vomiting and in many "love potions," and to treat infertile women. A part of Chinese medicine for more than 2,000 years, Chinese ginseng was used as an aphrodisiac	Boosts energy, fights debility, relieves hangovers, decreases blood pressure, relieves hot flashes, may reduce the risk of cancer, and may have anti-diabetic effects.

herb	historical use	present use
GINSENG *(cont.)*	and a painkiller, and to improve mental and physical vitality.	
LADY'S MANTLE	Used in medieval times to abate bleeding, especially in healing wounds and to ease menstruation. Also believed to aid in conception; women were instructed to bathe in water with this herb in order to retain the pregnancy.	Still used today to ease menstrual cramps; it has astringent properties, and may inhibit tumor growth.
LEMON BALM	For intestinal cramps and gas.	Relieves nervousness and insomnia.
MAY APPLE	The Cherokee used a juice derived from may apple root to cure deafness.	Wart removal.
MONKSHOOD	Was used externally for curing toothaches and sciatica. In Greek mythology, Medea is said to have poisoned Theseus with it.	Not used today, as it is poisonous.
PARSLEY	Parsley was widely used in teas as a digestive aid and to treat kidney stones.	For poor urine flow and kidney problems.

Herb	Historical use	Present use
Redcedar	Native Americans used tea made from this for worms, cold, coughs, and rheumatism.	Irritating to the skin, but can be used to treat warts and blisters. Today it is believed that this should not be taken internally.
Rosemary	In ancient times it was believed to improve memory and thereby encourage fidelity between lovers, and was used at weddings, funerals, and many religious ceremonies. Also used to purify the air at hospitals, expel bad dreams, remove hair, treat skin conditions, prevent tooth decay, and improve bad breath.	Cures headaches, acts as an astringent and stimulant, and prevents dandruff.
Salad burnet	American soldiers during the Revolutionary War drank salad burnet tea before battle to prevent excessive bleeding.	Heals wounds and sunburn.
Wild Ginger	Used in Chinese medicine for over 2,500 years primarily to purify the body through perspiration, to stimulate the appetite,	Treats loss of appetite and travel sickness.

Herb	Historical use	Present use
WILD GINGER *(cont.)*	and to calm nausea. In ayurvedic medicine, ginger has been used to treat arthritis. Native Americans used the juice of wild ginger root to keep snakes from biting.	
Yellow lady slipper	Popularly used in the nineteenth century to treat hysteria, insomnia, depression, and nerves.	Use today is not encouraged as it is strongly acidic and has a burning taste.

HOME REMEDIES

Creative home remedies have been passed down for generations, ranging from old favorites on how to cure hiccups to lesser-known tips on how to soothe engorged breasts. The origins of such treatments have been lost to time, and their actual effectiveness has been proved anecdotally. This listing is not intended be an endorsement of the treatments, and please do not use the remedies below without first consulting with your health-care provider.

- **Hiccups.** Drink a glass of water with a tablespoon of sugar. Sugar is believed to be an effective hiccup remedy because it has a relaxing effect on muscles.
- **Yeast and vaginal infections.** Douche with yogurt, which has antimicrobial properties.

- **Acne.** Put a lemon slice over the affected area for a few minutes. Alternatively, wrap an ice cube in a towel or cloth napkin and hold it against the affected area.
- **Baggy eyes.** Lie down and put a wet tea bag over your eyes. Relax for fifteen minutes. The tannin in the tea is an astringent and will help to firm up the baggy skin. You can also use cucumber slices instead of tea bags. Also, avoid salty foods the night before.
- **Belching.** In certain Asian cultures, belching is considered to be a compliment to the chef. But if your excessive burping is a social stigma where you come from, you might try chewing celery, anise, and fennel seeds (one variety at a time or mixed together) or ginger (see "Ginger" in the "Herbs in History" table). Also, try cutting down on carbonated drinks, hot, spicy foods, and onions.
- **Engorged breasts.** Women who are nursing or weaning often suffer from painfully engorged breasts. This happens when the supply of milk being produced exceeds the demand, creating a buildup. When nursing doesn't relieve this condition, a common treatment is the artful application of cabbage leaves. Women suffering from engorgement are often advised by their doctors, midwives, and lactation specialists, as well as by health books and Web sites, to take the following steps: (1) Wash several cabbage leaves, allow them to dry, and refrigerate them in plastic bags until needed. (2) Crumple the leaves to crush the veins. (3) Stuff the bra with the cabbage leaves until all the areas of the breasts are covered. (4) Apply new leaves in a couple of

hours, after the leaves begin to wilt. Several scientific studies have been conducted to determine how and why cabbage leaves help relieve engorgement. However, no definitive conclusions have been reached, and researchers are still at a loss to explain the mysterious curative effects of this cruciferous vegetable.

- **Flatulence.** Drink a teaspoon of apple cider vinegar with every meal.
- **Foot odor.** Mix two teaspoons of apple cider vinegar in a gallon of water. Soak your feet.
- **Headaches.** Take a lime, cut it in half, and rub it on the forehead.
- **Indigestion.** Try teas made from peppermint, chamomile, or catnip.
- **Motion sickness.** Drink some ginger tea or ginger ale, or chew on a piece of candied ginger.
- **Ulcers.** Drink cabbage juice. Cabbage is rich in the amino acid glutamine, which has healing properties.
- **Warts.** To treat a wart, take a small piece of ripe banana peel and place it over the wart, white side down. Tape the peel firmly in place and wear it all day. Change the peel each day after bathing. The chemicals in the peel will soften the wart and eventually kill it.

GEM THERAPY

Gem and crystal therapy have been part of healing traditions throughout the world, including those of the Chinese, Indian, Egyptian, and Jewish cultures. In the gem therapy tradition, semiprecious and precious stones are used for physical, spiritual, and mental healing, and much of the gems' powers are linked to their alignment with the planets. Our bodies are believed to have special energy channels called "meridians," and when energy movement along these channels becomes blocked or unbalanced, illness results. Diamonds, jade, and other stones are thought to store and generate electromagnetic energy that can correct these blockages and imbalances.

For centuries, priests, Buddhist monks, astrologers, and others have attributed mystical and curative powers to crystals and gemstones, and there are many recorded accounts of the use of gems in folk remedies. For example, there is a considerable amount of literature and lore on the healing powers of blue sapphires. According to the article "Sapphire: A Miracle Gem" by Dr. P. C. Lunia, a blue sapphire held against the temples was at one time believed to stop a nosebleed. Some believed that blue sapphires could not only heal sores but cause a carbuncle to discharge its poison with a single touch. A nineteenth-century occult writer named Francis Barrett declared that if a blue sapphire was rubbed on a new tumor, it would "draw out" the poison of the disease. In India and the Middle East, a blue sapphire was thought to provide the wearer with headache relief as well as protection against the evil eye.

Today, practitioners of crystal and gem therapy wear the stones, place them in their homes, and carry them around. Some concoct "elixirs" made with gems, as they did with topaz in the days of the great plague epidemics. The elixirs can be applied to the body, placed under the tongue with a dropper, or swallowed outright.

THE GOLDEN CURE

If you are looking for a free and readily available cure for your asthma, allergies, or acne problems, search no farther than the toilet. For centuries some Eastern and Western health practitioners have advocated the use of urine for medicinal purposes. This practice is known as "urine therapy" or "auto-urine therapy."

In urine therapy, one's own urine may be swallowed, applied to the skin, injected, sniffed, or used as an enema, as eyedrops, or as eardrops. Urine consists mostly of water plus small amounts of urea, salt, ammonia, and hundreds of other compounds. Proponents of urine therapy believe that it works by purifying the blood and tissues, allowing the body to "reabsorb" useful nutrients, hormones, enzymes, and other substances, thereby producing an autoimmunization effect similar to that provided by a vaccine.

To date, there have been no controlled scientific studies done to prove or disprove the effectiveness of urine therapy, and it is regarded by many with great skepticism. Still, urine therapy has been practiced in India for thousands of years and is widely used today in Hindu folk medicine. Advocates in India and elsewhere in the world claim that it can cure a range of ailments including colds, sore throats, asthma, allergies, skin conditions, ulcers, digestive problems, anorexia, alcoholism, and even cancer and AIDS.

The first World Conference on Urine Therapy was held in India in 1997, and the second in Germany in 1999. A third conference in Brazil is planned for the near future. According to the old Amsterdam-based Urinet Web site, which is devoted to the practice of urine therapy: "The international conference is meant to create a deeper understanding of the dynamics of urine therapy, to promote the use of urine therapy amongst doctors and health practitioners as well as the general public, and to exchange knowledge and experiences between urine therapy professionals."

Urine therapy has practitioners in the United States as well. An article in the August 2002 issue of *Cosmopolitan* magazine titled "6 Beauty Lies (and 5 Surprising Truths)" described urine as having moisturizing and acne-fighting properties. It pointed out that urea, a protein found in mammalian urine, is a common ingredient in many lotions. However, the urea found in cosmetics is not from human or animal urine; it's synthetically created.

MEDICAL INNOVATION

Serious medical conditions often leave communities puzzled for years, leading physicians and healers to try just about anything to cure them. Improvisation has led to some of the greatest medical discoveries in history, and in some cases *how* the remedies were found is more interesting than the remedies themselves. The innovative discoveries of the smallpox vaccine, insulin as a treatment for diabetes, and the mechanism of allergic reactions are a few examples that will be discussed in this chapter. We may now take these common treatments for granted, but when the experimentation that was involved in their discovery was undertaken, it was considered nothing short of radical.

HOLD THE BACON

Myiasis is a particularly unpleasant condition in which fly larvae penetrate human skin and live under the surface, breathing through an opening of the skin. Upon close inspection by the naked eye, the larvae can sometimes be seen wiggling around.

Because the larvae can burrow deeply, myiasis has been difficult to treat until recently. According to Robert M. Youngson's book *Medical Curiosities,* doctors at Boston's Massachusetts General Hospital discovered an effective new treatment in 1993. The treatment involved bacon, a favorite food of fly larvae. Pieces of raw bacon fat were applied to the skin. Within three hours, the larvae had emerged far enough to allow medical personnel to grab them with forceps and extract them. Youngson quoted an editor at the British medical journal *The Lancet* who had written about this technique: "The bacon should be discarded after use."

THE SMALLPOX VACCINE

In 1796 a British scientist and surgeon named Edward Jenner stumbled upon a vaccine for one of the deadliest diseases in history. Dr. Jenner was aware of a common but untested belief: that people who contracted cowpox never seemed to get

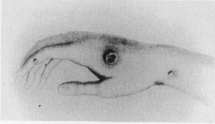

smallpox. Cowpox was a fairly benign illness that one could pick up easily from coming into contact with cows.

Dr. Jenner decided to conduct a risky experiment using a milkmaid named Sarah Nelmes who had cowpox lesions on her hand. Dr. Jenner took samples from one of the lesions and injected it into the skin of an eight-year-old boy named James Phipps. The boy suffered from a fever and other mild symptoms but otherwise did not become seriously ill.

Several weeks later—in a move that would appall people today but hardly raised eyebrows back in the eighteenth century—Dr. Jenner injected poor young James with the smallpox virus. Fortunately, James never came down with smallpox, and the smallpox vaccine, derived from human cowpox bacteria, was born.

THE NATURE OF ALLERGIES

According to Lexi Krock's *Nova Online* article "Accidental Discoveries," some credit for the modern treatment of allergies can go to a French physiologist named Charles Robert Richet, who lived from 1850 to 1935.

Richet was doing a series of experiments that involved exposing dogs to the poison from sea anemone tentacles. Not surprisingly, some of the dogs died after several days of allergy-related symptoms such as vomiting, shock, and loss of consciousness. But other dogs managed to survive the deadly treatments.

Several weeks later he injected the surviving dogs again. This time, not only did the dogs have allergic reactions to the poison but they had them within minutes—not days—of getting the injections. Several of them died almost immediately.

Richet realized that each time the dogs were exposed to the sea anemone poison, they reacted more severely. This led to his discovery of the mechanism of "anaphylaxis," as in *anaphylactic shock*. Richet postulated that the process of exposure to an allergen led to a gradual loss of immunity against, and an increased sensitivity to, that allergen. In 1913, Richet won the Nobel prize for this and other discoveries in the field of allergies and immunity.

INSULIN AND DIABETES

In 1923, Dr. Frederick G. Banting, a physician, and Professor John J. R. MacLeod of the University of Toronto shared the Nobel prize for Physiology or Medicine for isolating and using insulin in the treatment of diabetes. (Actually, MacLeod did none of the insulin work, and Banting was furious that Canadian physician Charles H. Best, his true partner in the insulin research, was passed over for the honor.)

MEDICINE IN THE WRONG HANDS

Today, insulin, a water-soluble hormone, is a godsend for diabetics. However, it can—in the wrong hands, under the wrong circumstances, or at the wrong doses—lead to "insulin shock": hypoglycemia (low blood sugar), nausea, vomiting, hypotension, shock, coma, and eventually death. Indeed, there are a number of murder-by-insulin cases in the record books. For example: According to a February 6, 2003, article by Matt Bean of CourtTV, Tonica Jenkins, a twenty-seven-year-old Cleveland-area woman, was arrested for the attempted murder of Melissa Latham. On April 21, 2001, Jenkins allegedly injected Latham with "catastrophic levels of insulin" in order to kill her; when that didn't quite do the job, Jenkins allegedly hired her cousin Kyle Martin to beat Latham with a brick.

Fortunately for Latham, Plan B didn't work, either. Left for dead, Latham managed to drag herself to a Kentucky Fried Chicken and get help.

According to Lexi Krock's "Accidental Discoveries" article, Banting's (and Best's) work would not have been possible without an accidental medical discovery many years before that. Krock wrote that in 1889, two German doctors, Joseph von Mering and Oscar Minkowski, wanted to study the connection between the pancreas and digestion. In order to do this, they removed the pancreas from a healthy dog but kept the dog alive. Several days later the doctors noticed that flies were swarming all over a puddle of the poor dog's urine. The doctors decided to test the urine and realized that it was full of sugar, which is a sign of diabetes. The doctors concluded that the dog had developed diabetes because it had lost its pancreas. They realized that a healthy pancreas was somehow responsible for secreting a substance that controlled sugar levels in the body. Some of the details of this story may or may not be legend, but the fact remains: Once again, an accidental discovery led to a significant medical breakthrough that would improve the lives of millions of people.

3. Parasites and Other Unwelcome Guests

Almost all the world is little else in nature but parasites or sub-parasites.

—Ben Jonson

The word *infestation* never denotes a good thing. There are no such things as *positive* infestations—say, an infestation of stock dividends or an infestation of attractive, interesting single people at a party. When we talk about infestations, we're usually talking about fleas, roaches, rodents, and other undesirable little creatures. And then there are even more loathsome and much smaller creatures that infest—in fact, you may be infested by a family of them right now and not even know it. Some of these creatures like to reside on your person; some of them, *in* your person.

Welcome to the world of parasites.

Most of us probably don't give a thought to parasites. We tend to believe that parasites happen in faraway places to other people—Third World countries with substandard sanitary conditions or economically challenged families with bad grooming habits.

Parasites may be more prevalent in these groups, but the rest of us probably could stand to lose a little sleep over the matter too. According to Ann Louise Gittleman's eye-opening (and stomach-turning) book *Guess What Came to Dinner? Parasites and Your Health,* "Americans today are host to more than 130 different kinds of parasites, ranging from microscopic organisms to foot-long tapeworms." In fact, some experts believe parasites to be a silent epidemic affecting millions of Americans and resulting in a variety of medical conditions—everything from fatigue to cancer. According to Gittleman's book, some scientists have even suggested that there may be a link between parasites and AIDS. For example, in amebiasis, an infection caused by amoebic cysts that have been ingested via contaminated food or water, immune defense cells can be destroyed that normally would engulf HIV, thus allowing the virus to spread throughout the body.

In this chapter you will learn about how parasites, from pinworms to lice, have infested human populations throughout history, and about some of the nastiest cases of parasites that have plagued the human body.

A BRIEF, UNPLEASANT GUIDE
TO PARASITES

Parasites are organisms ranging in size from microscopic on up that require a living host for their survival. Acording to

Gittleman, parasites are "categorized according to structure, shape, function, and reproductive ability." These categories include Nematoda (roundworms, pinworms, and hookworms), Cestoda (tapeworms), Trematoda (flukes), and Protozoa (single-celled microscopic organisms).

Parasites will invade their host and settle into the intestines or migrate elsewhere within the body. Parasites often enter the host via the skin, the mouth, or the bottoms of the feet. They can be found in a variety of places, including meat, vegetables, soil, and feces. Their eggs or larvae can be ingested in contaminated foods that are uncooked or undercooked. The eggs can also become airborne and be ingested via the respiratory system.

Parasitic infestations may or may not result in symptoms. The presence and type of symptoms will depend on the type and extent of the infestation; a few of the possible symptoms include diarrhea, abdominal pain, nausea, dysentery, weight loss, and anemia. The symptoms can range from mild to life-threatening, and the worms may go undetected for a long time. They may also be seen in one's fecal matter.

We know from fossilized feces found by archaeologists that parasites have a long, proud history of bothering humans. Archaeologists who study the fossilized feces of humans and animals can actually reconstruct the medical history of ancient societies on the basis of the kinds of parasites found in their fecal waste. By analyzing these worms, scientists can determine what kinds of foods people were eating and how different diseases evolved and spread throughout communities.

According to pathoecologist Karl Reinhard in an interview with *Discover* magazine, one factor that led to the increase in parasite infestations was urbanization. In hunter-gatherer societies, parasite infestations were minor and came mostly from eating insects. But as people came to live closer together, they gained not only each other as neighbors but parasites as well. This was partially due to the fact that their fecal matter was now concentrated in one place rather than spread out over a vast area. Reinhard said that when a Pueblo group known as the Anasazi Indians began creating villages in caves approximately 10,000 years ago, the level of pinworm infection approached 100 percent.

Reinhard went on to explain that when communities began settling along rivers, this led to an increase in parasites such as whipworms, roundworms, and hookworms, presumably because these rivers became contaminated with fecal matter. In a related article, "Mummy's Ruin? Health Hazards and Cures in Ancient Egypt," author Joyce M. Filer wrote that when Egyptians settled on the banks of the river Nile they used its water for drinking, cooking, and washing. But the standing water in the river's irrigation channels was also a breeding ground for parasites. These parasites probably entered the bodies of people through their feet and legs as they waded in the water; the parasites then laid eggs in the humans' bloodstreams. When these eggs hatched, the parasites could travel to different organs, causing great damage and making the human hosts more susceptible to disease.

Another historical factor that led to the increase in parasite infestations was the domestication of animals. This paved the way for a phenomenon known as "host-jumping," in which parasites that traditionally infected only animals were able to jump on over to humans.

According to Karl Reinhard, the building of adobe houses was yet another historical development that led to a particularly terrible parasitic disease. Chagas' disease is caused by a protozoan that enters the intestinal tract and causes people to stop excreting. The protozoan in question happens to love adobe houses, and was not around before people started building them. Scientists have discovered mummies with fecal masses "the size of soccer balls" in their intestines, said Reinhard. Unable to eliminate, these people would have died slow, painful deaths. Chagas' disease is unfortunately still around today, mostly in South America.

Studies and anecdotal evidence suggest that a majority of Americans may have some kind of parasite in their bodies. They can be a serious problem, especially for children, whose immune systems are more sensitive than those of adults. In his introduction to *Guess What Came to Dinner?* Dr. Omar M. Amin wrote that approximately fifty million American children are estimated to have some type of worm parasite infection.

Such factors as international travel, the increased risk to children presented by daycare centers, and contaminated water sources have contributed to the spread of parasites. Pets also contribute to the problem, since they are common carriers of parasites. According to Gittleman in her book, there are 240 infectious diseases that can pass from animals to humans, and of these, cats are responsible for 39 of them, and dogs, 65. Children, pregnant women, and immunocompromised people are particularly vulnerable to such parasitic infections as dog and cat roundworm, dog and cat hookworm, and cat-transmitted toxoplasmosis.

Gruesome anecdotal accounts of modern-day parasitic infestation abound. One woman reportedly passed more than three cups of hookworms—all six inches long and gray—while having a colonic treatment to clean out her colon. Another woman sought help because she kept seeing "rainbows" every

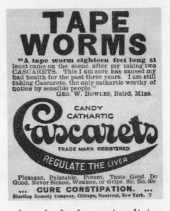

time the sun was out; it turned out that she had parasites living in the retinas of her eyes. Yet another woman found tiny maggotlike parasites in the water when she got up out of her bath; the same parasites showed up when she urinated into her toilet.

There are awful, and more substantiated, parasite stories as well. According to various AP, ABC News, and other news reports summarized in a Web site article called "It Could Happen to You or Someone You Love," in 1993, 400,000 residents of Milwaukee got sick, and 100 died, from parasites in the water supply. In 1994 a mysterious tapewormlike parasite invaded a man's abdomen, destroyed three fourths of his liver, and eventually killed him. In 1997 a tapeworm got into the brain of a ten-year-old California boy, triggering a seizure. A parasite called *Pfiesteria piscicida*, dubbed the "cell from hell," killed tens of thousands of fish from Delaware to Alabama and affected human swimmers as well. In 1996 and 1997, more than a thousand Americans grew sick from the parasite *Cayetanensis cyclospora*, mostly from outbreaks traced to consumption of raspberries from Guatemala, lettuce, and possibly basil.

Still, in a majority of the reported cases, parasitic worm infestations tend to be more common in areas of the world with low hygienic standards. If you happen to be in those parts—or even if you're not—here are some general ground rules for avoiding contamination:

- Do not go to the bathroom outdoors.
- Avoid contact with soil that may be contaminated with animal or human waste.
- Dispose of diapers in proper hygienic fashion.
- Wash hands thoroughly with soap and water after going to the bathroom.
- Wash hands thoroughly with soap and water before handling food.
- Wash, peel, or cook all raw veggies and fruits before eating.
- If you happen to find yourself in a country where sanitation and hygiene are less than ideal, avoid eating food that may be contaminated. Avoid drinking or bathing in water that may be contaminated.

If you *do* succumb, the best treatment is a hasty visit to your doctor and, most likely, prescription medication. Unfortunately, worm infestations can be difficult to detect in the early stages and difficult to treat once entrenched. Some but not all worms like to live in the intestines for a time.

Here is a sampling of the more common parasites that like to share space with humans and other hosts.

A NOTE TO MALE READERS

According to a September 20, 2002, article on the *Scientific American* Web site, a study by the University of Stirling in Scotland shows that parasites seem to have a distinct preference for the males of a number of species. This "preferential treatment" results in higher death rates from parasitic infection for males. The study authors suggest that "male machismo" may be the reason for this phenomenon: Parasites may be more attracted to the larger bodies of males. Researchers from other universities acknowledged that this could hold true for humans as well. In fact, even in countries with sophisticated medical care (e.g., the United States), men are twice as likely as females to die from parasitic diseases such as malaria.

PINWORMS

These little fellows—also known as *Enterobius vermicularis*—are, unfortunately, very common parasites in the United States. Infestation can happen if one happens to ingest the worm eggs via food, water, household dust, or by coming into contact with an infected human. Once swallowed, the worm eggs become big grown-up worms that live in your intestines. In the evenings the female worms will crawl out of your anus in order to lay eggs in the anal area. This can cause intense itching (as well as the overwhelming urge to burn your sheets and pajamas, then take a three-hour-long hot shower while muttering insanely like Lady Macbeth). Once in a while the tiny white worms are visible in the feces after a number two. You can tell them apart from any other white matter in your feces because they will be wriggling.

HOOKWORMS

Imagine a worm that attaches itself to your intestinal wall with hooklike teeth and sucks your blood. This is the noble hookworm, aka *Necator americanus* and *Ancylostoma duodenale.*

Hookworm larvae live in soil and can actually penetrate human skin. The larvae take a little trip through the bloodstream to the lungs and windpipe and then settle in the intestines, where they grow up into adult worms and play Dracula with your blood.

Hookworm is more common in tropical countries than in the United States. If you live in the United States, try not to walk barefoot through sewage-contaminated water, which is the number-one method of contracting hookworm in this country.

According to Gittleman's book, "hookworms can live up to fifteen years in the human body."

TOXOCARIASIS

Many a horrified parent has come upon his or her baby grabbing playfully at the contents of the litter box. Here is one more reason not to let the little ones indulge in that bad habit: toxocariasis.

The *Toxocara canis* and *Toxocara cati* roundworms like to infest our pet dogs and cats. When our pets go to the litter box or out into the yard, the roundworm eggs get excreted along with the, um, excreta. If we happen to touch this excreta (or litter or soil contaminated by it) and then are unwise enough to touch our mouths or the like, we will become similarly infested with *Toxocara* eggs. The eggs hatch in our intestines, blossom into larvae, then travel to other parts of our bodies: lungs, liver, and sometimes eyes (where they can cause temporary or permanent blindness) and brain (where they can cause epilepsy).

If you suspect that you have toxocariasis, see your doctor promptly. A blood test will tell you if that's what ails you. Toxocariasis is treatable with medication; in the rare instances in which it spreads to the eye, it can be more difficult to treat, and medical measures must be employed to prevent progressive eye damage.

Ascariasis

Ascariasis is an infection caused by the ascarid worm living in your small intestine. Female ascarid worms can grow up to twelve inches in length; males tend to be smaller.

Ascariasis is the most common human worm infection in the world. Approximately one in four people will have this infestation at some time in their life. Infection is rare in the United States; when it happens, it tends to happen in rural areas of the Southeast. Ascariasis is most common in tropical and subtropical countries with poor sanitation and hygiene. Ascarisis can strike you but lead to no symptoms whatsoever. With a serious infection, abdominal pain can occur, as can intestinal blockage. If the immature worms travel through your lungs, you may develop a cough or other respiratory problems.

As for the hard facts: The usual method of ascariasis infestation is eating contaminated food or drinking contaminated beverages. Bad hygiene, bad sanitation, and use of human fecal matter as fertilizer are contributing causes. Fertilizer made from pig feces is another concern. Pigs can be infected with ascarids and can pass their infection on to humans if their contaminated fecal matter happens to be used to fertilize crops. So when you're putting in your vegetable garden next year, stick to Miracle-Gro!

Diagnosis of ascariasis can be made with a stool sample brought to your doctor. If you happen to cough up a worm or pass one in your stool, be sure to bring him/her along as well. (This is not a joke: It can happen.) The usual treatment is a round of medication.

TRICHINOSIS

According to the Centers for Disease Control and Prevention Web site, in 1995 a man shot and killed a cougar near Elk City, Idaho. He took the unfortunate cat home and made jerky out of it. (Recipe for all you gourmands out there: Soak the cougar meat in a brine solution made from table salt, then smoke in smoker.) Unfortunately, the man's smoker never reached the desired smoking temperature—above "warm." But the man chowed down on the jerky anyway, and also distributed the meat to fourteen other lucky people.

Within weeks, the man came down with trichinosis. So did nine of the fourteen jerky recipients. The jerky was examined at the Sacred Heart Medical Center in Spokane, Washington, and found to contain *Trichinella spiralis* larvae.

Not to be confused with trikona-asana (the triangle posture in yoga) or trichotillomania (a compulsive hair-pulling disorder), trichinosis, also called trichinellosis, is a wicked infection caused by the *T. spiralis* worm. The culprit is usually undercooked pork or wild game products that happen to contain larval stages of this worm, which are encapsulated; the larval capsules are called cysts.

The initial symptoms of trichinosis, which can appear one to two days after ingestion of the contaminated meat, include abdominal discomfort, nausea, vomiting, diarrhea, fatigue, and fever. The second set of symptoms, which can take two to eight weeks to surface, include muscle pains, aching joints, headache, fever, chills, cough, swelling of the eyes, itchy skin, and constipation (or, conversely, more diarrhea). In serious cases, trichinosis can lead to complications such as acute heart failure or a meningitis-like condition. In severe cases, trichinosis can be fatal. The severity of the case will depend mainly on the number of worms originally ingested. If the case is extremely mild, it can go away on its own; people may even attribute the symptoms to the flu or other passing illness. You will be at risk for this infection if you eat raw or undercooked meats, particularly pork, bear, wild cats, dog, horse, fox, wolf, seal, or walrus.

Here is a historical case in point. In 1897 an explorer named Salomon August Andree led an expedition to the Arctic in a balloon. He and two other men wanted to be the first ones to cross the North Pole. Unfortunately, during the journey the balloon experienced a number of problems, and the men were forced to land. Legend has it that the men were in despair until they shot and killed a polar bear. Now the men had real food!

Years later, the three men's skeletons were discovered by a ship's crew. From the descriptions in Andree's diaries, it appeared that the men had died from trichinosis contracted from raw polar-bear meat.

Fortunately, smart people these days know better than to eat raw polar-bear meat or undersmoke the cougar. Still, those who suspect trichinosis need to get to a doctor ASAP for a blood test or muscle biopsy.

Here are some ways recommended by the Centers for Disease Control to avoid contracting trichinosis:

- Cook all meat and meat products to an internal temperature of 170 degrees Fahrenheit, or until the juices run clear.
- Freeze pork and pork products less than six inches thick for twenty days at 5 degrees Fahrenheit to kill any worms.
- Freezing wild-game meats, even for long periods of time, may not necessarily kill worms. You must cook them thoroughly.
- Do not eat meat from livestock or wild animals that may have eaten raw or undercooked meat, including rat carcasses, which can be infected with trichinosis.
- If you prepare your own ground meats, clean the meat grinders thoroughly.

- Note that curing (salting), drying, smoking, or micro-waving meat does not guarantee that infectious worms will be thoroughly killed.

TAPEWORMS

Maria Callas, the renowned opera diva, subjected herself to all kinds of crash diets and diuretics in order to correct her famous "weight problem." At the end of 1953, she finally began to make a dent. Over the next few years she lost a whopping 66 pounds, going from 210 to 144 pounds. Her beauty secret? A tapeworm infestation. While this fact is vigorously debated on various "urban legend" Web sites, the point is still well taken. Tapeworms can lead to dramatic weight loss, among other things.

There are three main varieties of large tapeworms that like to colonize humans and help them eat their food for them: the fish tapeworm (*Diphyllobothrium latum*), beef tapeworm (*Taenia saginata*), and pork tapeworm (*T. solium*). As you might expect, the most common cause of infestation is eating raw or under-cooked meat or fish containing larvae. Once in your tummy, the little creatures grow up into big adults. They can some-times reach twenty to thirty feet in length, or even longer.

Tapeworms are very efficient creatures. Being hermaph-roditic, they actually manage to fertilize themselves, as they have both testes and ovaries in each segment of their long, flat bodies. A fish tapeworm, which can consist of thousands of segments, is capable of producing more than 1 million eggs a day.

If you are cursed with a beef or pork tapeworm, you may feel an increase in appetite: After all, you are eating for two! With the beef tapeworm, you may feel segments of the creature wriggling out of your anus. This is a sure way of diagnosing the problem, since at this point you will probably be running, screaming in horror, to your doctor. Fortunately, tapeworm infestation can be cured with a single dose of an anthelmintic, or worm-expelling, drug.

There are many legends regarding gruesomely long tapeworms residing inside humans. By several accounts, the longest tapeworm passed by a human being was 33 meters, or 108 feet. The author was not able to authenticate this story or find the identity of the lucky person. However, there was an interesting story floating around on several Web sites regarding a Ms. Sally Mae Wallace of Great Grits, Mississippi, who believed *she* held the tapeworm record. On September 5, 1991, doctors apparently extracted 37 continuous feet of tapeworm from Ms. Wallace. Said she: "About after twenty feet of that thing had come out of my mouth, I just knew I had the record. I was really filled with joy."

SCHISTOSOMIASIS

A fluke is not just a "chance occurrence." It's also a type of tapeworm that can cause a nasty condition known as schistosomiasis. It is transmitted to humans by means of freshwater snails.

Schistosomiasis tends to affect people who ingest the snails while swimming or wading in lakes, canals, or unchlorinated pools, mainly in developing countries. Several hundred million people are believed to be contaminated with it worldwide. It is not found in the United States. Symptoms include "swimmer's itch" at the point where the fluke entered the skin, as well as fever, muscle pains, diarrhea, and more. If the fluke penetrates the bladder or liver, it can cause long-term damage to those organs.

If you find yourself in a country where schistosomiasis occurs and your skin comes in contact with fresh water from canals, rivers, streams, or lakes, you may be at risk of contracting an infection. The best prevention is to avoid swimming or wading in fresh water in those countries. Chlorinated swimming pools and the ocean are generally thought to be safe. Drinking water must also be made safe, by either boiling or filtering.

If you think you have been infected, get to a doctor. A blood or stool sample will provide a diagnosis. There are safe medications to treat schistosomiasis.

To end on a bright note: Flukes are proof that there is love even within the parasite kingdom. The adults of the schistosomiasis flukes live in pairs, with the female fluke residing cozily in a groove in the male fluke's body.

HYDATID DISEASE

Do not feed your dog raw offal. It can give you hydatid disease. (In case you are wondering what hydatid disease is, it is characterized by hydatid cysts, filled with cells that can grow into worms. They may be present in infected offal. In case you are wondering what offal is, it's the waste parts of slaughtered animals, especially sheep.)

This is how it works: If your dog happens to eat raw offal that happens to contain tapeworm larvae, its intestines will become a breeding ground for adult tapeworms. When the poor pup poops, tapeworm eggs will be passed out.

Then, if the eggs happen to enter your person (via your mouth, if you are not a good and thorough hand washer), they will move into your intestines and hatch into larvae. The larvae will proceed to journey merrily through your body, causing pain and jaundice and other unpleasant symptoms.

GIARDIASIS

Let's get off the topic of worms and discuss a few other parasitic creatures. For example, there is a tiny, tiny parasite called *Giardia lamblia* that can be ingested by drinking contaminated water (beware, hikers and campers!) or observing poor hygiene while hanging out with *Giardia*-infected animals, particularly dogs and beavers.

The good news is that giardiasis is treatable with antibiotics. The bad news is that the infection can recur. The other bad news is that one of the symptoms of giardiasis is excessive belching and farting. Not a pretty illness!

HEAD LICE

Parents of school-age children are all too familiar with a parasite known as the head louse (plural: head lice). Lice are tiny creatures that attach themselves to the scalp, feed on human blood, and lay tiny eggs, or "nits." The primary symptom of a lice infestation is very bad itching. Lice can be easily transmitted from person to person through close contact, sharing of combs or brushes, or sleeping on the same sheets.

There are many remedies for head lice: chemical or homeopathic poisons to kill the lice; a solution that causes lice to glow in the dark, making them easier to spot and remove; and even professional delousers who will come to your house and comb the critters out. Some experts recommend aromatic lice killers such as the essential oils of tea tree, cinnamon, rosemary, and oregano.

Lice are not new to society. Societies as long ago as ancient Egypt suffered greatly from lice infestations. We even have the evidence: Remains of head lice have been found in ancient Egyptians tombs along with artifacts such as jewels, scarabs, and mummies.

And for as long as there have been lice, there have existed remedies whose purpose was to get rid of them. According to "A Problem as Old as the Pyramids," a Web site article by Judith Illes, one ancient Egyptian remedy for removing lice was a warm potion of date meal and water. Egyptian men and women also routinely shaved their heads in an effort to keep the little guys away. The beautiful hairstyles ancient Egyptians are remembered for were the result of wigs, which Egyptians were very fond of for aesthetic as well as health reasons. A rich Egyptian woman might own many wigs in many different styles, lengths, and colors, complete with carrying cases. Her own head was shaved to control lice.

Indeed, the Egyptians were very creative about pest control. According to Illes's article, other Egyptian remedies against vermin include spreading cats' fat all over everything, to keep mice away, and sprinkling a solution of natron in water around the home, to keep fleas away. While we sincerely hope that cats' fat is no longer used for this purpose, sprinkling salt on carpets and then vacuuming is a method still used to combat fleas.

A variation on the theme of head lice is pubic lice, a.k.a. crabs. They will hang out in your pubic hair and, like head lice, feed on your blood and lay nits. The nits attach themselves so firmly to the pubic hair that bathing, even in scalding water, even screaming "Die, vermin!" will not wash them away.

Pubic lice are usually spread via sexual contact. Symptoms include major itching in the pubic and anal regions, especially at night. Another way to know that you are infected is to actually see the nits or grown-up lice crawling around Down There.

PARASITOSIS

In her Web site article "Bug Off," Barbara Boughton described a woman with an unusual problem. The woman came to see a doctor, complaining of parasites. She sat down and began pulling little things out of her nose. "These are the parasites that are bothering me," she said in a distressed voice. "They're crawling inside my nose."

The doctor studied the parasites under a microscope. He told her that they were not parasites but bits of Kleenex.

They were parasites, the patient insisted.

The woman was suffering from a delusional disorder known as parasitosis. With parasitosis, a person imagines that his or her body has been invaded by parasites, including worms, insects, fleas, and mites. People suffering from this condition often deliver or mail little containers to doctors full of the so-called parasites in hopes of getting treatment. Some will go from doctor to doctor, hoping to find one who will "cure" them of their infestation.

According to Boughton, when two scientists published a paper about the strange new tapewormlike parasite that had killed an AIDS patient in 1994, they were besieged with calls, letters, and e-mails from people who seemed to be suffering from parasitosis. These people claimed that they, too, had the mysterious new parasite; some claimed that their bodies were absolutely teeming with them.

Another woman suffering from parasitosis complained that her body and surroundings were being overrun by bugs. She said that bugs were crawling out of her scalp and drinking out of her eyes.

Another parasitosis victim—a man—thought that he had parasites that were secreting a substance all over his house. The substance was oily and amber-colored, the man claimed. It coated his skin, covered the walls of his home, and gummed up his washer and dryer.

PARASITE REMOVAL

A number of remedies have been used throughout history to combat different types of pesky parasites. Some of them are still in use today. Here are some examples from Ann Gittleman's book *Guess What Came to Dinner?* But please note that they are for your reading pleasure only! If you think you have a parasite infestation, see your doctor first and foremost. According to Gittleman, even "home remedies" should be used in conjunction with a health care practitioner's care.

To cleanse the intestines of parasites: rice bran fiber, psyllium seed fiber, flaxseed fiber, alfalfa leaves, fennel seed, anise seed, butternut root bark, buckthorn bark, licorice root, Irish moss, apple pectin, or citrus pectin.

For home enemas: garlic, vinegar, blackstrap molasses, or coffee mixed with milk or water.

For a parasite-unfriendly diet: pineapples, pomegranate juice, papaya seeds or papayas, pumpkinseeds, raw garlic, onions, radishes, raw cabbage, sauerkraut, kelp, fig extract, ground almonds, blackberries, lemon seeds, mugwort tea, or Corsican seaweed tea.

Some parasite-unfriendly herbs (for cooking or ingesting via tinctures, capsules, or powders) are: peppermint leaves, wormwood, pinkroot, goldenseal, sage, cloves, tansy, thyme, cranberry powder, oil of oregano, and male fern.

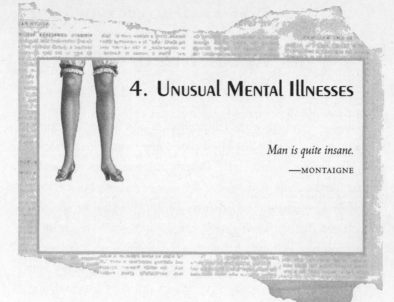

4. Unusual Mental Illnesses

Man is quite insane.

—MONTAIGNE

THE MIND IS A DARK AND MYSTERIOUS PLACE. WE ALL know this, and know, directly or indirectly, the effects of mental illness—for example, not being able to get out of bed, drinking to excess, sabotaging relationships, or crying too much.

As if those symptoms weren't bad enough, there are a number of mental illnesses out there that make everyday depression seem like a day at the beach. Some of them are delusional disorders that make a person think he or she is someone (or something) else entirely. Some of the disorders involve compulsive, uncontrollable behavior. Still other disorders lead their victims to commit acts of brutal violence against themselves and others.

Here is a smattering of these disorders, many of which continue to confuse and plague the experts.

THE STRANGE CASE OF THE WALKING CORPSE

A man diagnosed with schizophrenia continued to stump his doctors when he displayed symptoms that did not exactly fit the schizophrenia "bill." Despite treatment, he repeatedly attempted suicide, had strange delusions and visual perception problems, and displayed other mysterious physical symptoms.

Upon further investigation, the doctors got to the root of his problem. The man believed—*truly believed*—that he was a walking corpse. He said he was dead because his family had killed him several years ago. As further proof of his nonliving state, the man reported that he *felt* dead, that he could not see as he used to when he was alive—for example, he could not see his feet while walking. He explained that his multiple attempts at suicide were meant to prove to everyone that he was, indeed, dead.

The man was diagnosed with Cotard syndrome, and his story is chronicled in a Web site article called "The Cotard Syndrome." Cotard syndrome is characterized by the delusional belief that one is a walking corpse. Also referred to as Cotard delusion, delirium of total negation, delusion of negation, and delusional nihilism, this strange ailment was named after Jules Cotard, who is credited with first describing it in 1890.

There are a number of ways in which victims of Cotard syndrome experience being dead while alive. They may believe that some or all of their internal organs—brain, heart, stomach, and so forth—are missing. They may think that their bodies have been reduced to machines, that they have turned to stone, or that they have been replaced by an empty shell. They may believe themselves to be stinking, rotting cadavers and feel worms crawling through their bodies (similar to what those suffering from cocaine or amphetamine psychosis can go through). Some may even request, or adamantly insist on, burial. Accord-

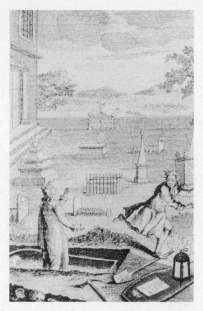

ing to one neurology and language Web site, a French physician named Charles Bonnet documented the case of a woman who insisted on being buried in a coffin. When her request was refused, she simply put herself in her coffin and lay there until she died a few weeks later.

Paradoxically, those suffering from Cotard syndrome might suddenly feel immortal, as if their bodies are expanding infinitely into space or that they can literally touch the stars. Other symptoms of Cotard syndrome can include anxiety, depression, difficulty recognizing people or places, paranoia, and catatonia. Reported treatments have included antidepressants and electroshock therapy.

As for the above-mentioned man who thought he was a walking corpse: In 1999 he received a series of twelve electroshock therapy treatments. As of early 2003 he was reported to be doing well and had not made any more suicide attempts.

THE OTHER

"S.M." had been deaf since she was five years old. In her seventies, she began doing sign language in front of mirrors. When asked to whom she was signing, she replied that she was signing to "the other S.M." She added that "the other S.M." was identical to her in all aspects, including her deafness—except that "the other S.M." was not as smart as she was.

S.M. was suffering from Capgras' syndrome, according to John Shea's article "The Fragile Orchestra." Capgras' syndrome is also known as delusional misidentification, illusion of doubles, illusion of negative doubles, misidentification syndrome, nonrecognition syndrome, phantom double syndrome, and subjective doubles syndrome. This disorder can cause a wife to point an accusing finger at her spouse and scream, "What have you done with my husband?"—and really mean it. It can also, as in the case of S.M., make the patient think that he or she is his or her own double. The misidentification can extend to objects: A Capgras' patient might believe that his watch or glasses have been replaced by a duplicate.

Capgras' syndrome was named after a turn-of-the-century French psychiatrist named Jean Marie Joseph Capgras (or perhaps his evil twin or an impostor). Some people theorize that Capgras' syndrome might provide a psychiatric explanation for reports of "alien abductions." (Remember *The Invasion of the Body Snatchers*?) There have also been recent incidents of Capgras' syndrome in which the patient believed that the Anti-christ had reappeared.

Capgras' syndrome can be accompanied by asomatognosia, which means "lack of recognition of the body." Patients suffering from this characteristic do not recognize parts of their own bodies and will go to the extent of disavowing or disowning them. They will even make up elaborate stories to explain the existence of these mysterious body parts.

There are several poignant examples of this in John Shea's article. In one case, a sixty-four-year-old construction worker had a stroke, and his left arm was left paralyzed as a result. The patient denied that he was sick, however, and even denied that he was in the hospital, even though he was. The patient told his doctor that it was his *mother* who was in the hospital (even though she wasn't). When his doctor indicated the patient's left arm and asked him what it was, the patient responded: "My mother-in-law's hand. Someone's hand."

Shea describes another case in which an elderly woman's left arm had been likewise paralyzed by a stroke. In the hospital the woman continued to insist that her left arm was not her left arm but her doctor's hand. She also referred to her left arm as a "breast" or as "deodorant." Furthermore, she told her doctor that her dead husband had bequeathed his hands to her in his will. "He just left them like he left his clothes," she explained. She added that she had recently thrown his hands away, just as she had done with his now-useless clothes.

FOLIE À DEUX

A man who suffered from alcoholism repeatedly sought the services of prostitutes. When his wife found out, he developed paranoid delusions that the prostitutes were following him in cars, calling him at home, spying on him on the street, and taking what little money he had left. (In reality, his illicit habits had greatly depleted the family savings.)

The wife, who had no previous history of mental illness, became convinced of the truth of his delusional beliefs. Together they kept an eye out for suspicious prostitutes and reported their behavior to local police as "harassment."

Shortly thereafter, the wife became even more ill and delusional. She believed that prostitutes were coming into her house; she was convinced they intended to humiliate her or hurt her. She made plans for her husband to kidnap a police officer for ransom. She then persuaded her husband to blow up a building that supposedly housed the prostitutes in question. He was caught and arrested while attempting to blow up the building.

According to the article "Shared Psychotic Disorder" by Dr. Sharon Idan and Eliyahu Yona, which describes this case at length, the husband was treated successfully for paranoid schizophrenia. The wife was diagnosed with folie à deux, literally, "double madness."

Folie à deux is a rare delusional disorder in which a submissive *nonpsychotic* person assumes the delusions of a dominant *psychotic* person with whom he or she has a close relationship. The delusions tend to be less far-fetched than in other types of psychoses—for example, delusions of persecution or sickness as opposed to, say, delusions of having been replaced by an alien life form. The submissive partner will truly assume—not just *pretend* to assume—the delusions of the dominant one in order to please the person, and because there is such a strong emotional connection between them. Sometimes called "shared delusional disorder," folie à deux strikes women more than men.

There are a number of bizarre cases of this disorder in the literature. Twins are common victims of this illness. Anecdotal evidence suggests that the identical twins Steven and Cyril Marcus, two New York physicians who became recluses and committed suicide together in 1975, may have suffered from folie à deux. The Marcus twins were the basis of the novel *Twins* by Bari Wood and Jack Geasland, which in turn was the basis of the David Cronenberg film *Dead Ringers.*

Folie à deux usually involves a person-to-person dynamic. But in one documented case, described by Robert Howard in the March 1992 issue of *The American Journal of Psychiatry*, the folie à deux occurred between a woman and her dog. In this case, the latter apparently shared the delusions of the former. The woman in question, an 83-year-old widow, complained that the man in the apartment above her was very noisy. She claimed that he moved furniture around in the middle of the night in order to bother her. Over time, the poor widow developed delusions about her upstairs neighbor. She believed that he was transmitting "violet rays" through the ceiling in order to hurt her and her pet dog. In fact, the widow blamed a sprained back and chest pains on the violet rays. She also claimed that her dog had begun scratching a lot at night, when the rays were at their most potent. She decided to protect herself by placing her mattress under the kitchen table and sleeping there. Likewise, she made what she referred to as an "air-raid shelter" for her dog with suitcases and a table, and she ordered the dog to sleep in it. As with classic folie à deux, the dog apparently began to share the delusions of its owner. Whenever the dog heard any sound from the upstairs apartment at all, it would immediately rush to its "air-raid shelter."

Folie à deux is often treated with therapy and medication—when the patients are human, anyway. In the real-life case of the wife of the man who liked prostitutes, however, she refused hospitalization and stopped taking her medications. At last report, she was still having delusions.

Strangely, folie à deux can sometimes be folie à trois, folie à quatre, or even more. There are reports of cases of multiple individuals being involved in shared delusions; there is even a case in which twelve family members were affected, a variation known as folie à famille. Some experts believe that folie à famille may be an operative factor in the behavior of members of cults such as the People's Temple (Jonestown), the Branch Davidians (Waco), and Aum Shinrikyo (Japan).

Indeed, folie à famille was evoked in the infamous Charles Manson case. Allegedly motivated by the Book of Revelations, the Beatles' song "Helter Skelter," and a need to "instill fear into the Establishment," Charles Manson and his "family" of followers brutally slaughtered Sharon Tate, the wife of film director Roman Polanski (she was eight months pregnant at the time), and four of her houseguests in the summer of 1969. They then went on to kill supermarket-chain owner

Leno LaBianca, and his wife, Rosemary, with kitchen utensils and various other gruesome tools.

Manson and his accomplices were convicted; however, one of the accomplices, Leslie Van Houten, who had been homecoming princess of Monrovia High School in Monrovia, California, received a retrial in 1976 because her lawyer had "disappeared" during the first trial. (His remains were found months later in the wilderness; some believe that he was murdered by someone in the Manson group, though this was never proved.) Van Houten's retrial in 1976 went awry for the prosecution because the defense claimed that Van Houten had suffered from "diminished capacity" in the form of folie à famille, and there was a hung jury. Van Houten was subsequently convicted in a third trial in 1978.

FATAL ATTRACTION

A psychiatrist named Doreen Orion found herself the object of one patient's passion. The patient, whom the doctor called "Fran," was convinced that Orion was in love with her, and was clearly puzzled when Orion responded to her overtures of love with restraining orders and threats to send Fran to jail. Fran continued to pursue, stalk, and harass Orion for eight years, obsessed with the idea that she had to bring Orion around to the "truth" of their mutual passion.

Fran suffered from erotomania, a mental disorder in which a person, often a woman, develops the delusional belief that a certain person is in love with her. Other names for this peculiar disorder include Clérambault's (or de Clérambault's) syndrome, Simenon's syndrome, erotic delusion, paranoia erotica, pure erotomania, and *psychose passionelle.*

With this disorder, the love object—who is often older and more prominent socially, professionally, or otherwise—is likely to be a distant acquaintance who has done nothing to encourage a romantic relationship. Furthermore, the love object is unaware of the delusion until he or she begins to receive phone calls, e-mails, and other correspondences along the lines of "You love me, I know you love me, *you can't hide it from me anymore.*" Criminal or borderline criminal behavior such as stalking, harassment, and even violence can occur. It is important to note that not all stalkers are erotomaniacs.

According to Katherine Ramsland's CourtTV article "All About Stalkers," celebrities are common targets of erotomaniacs. In 1989 the twenty-one-year-old actress Rebecca Schaeffer, star of the sitcom *My Sister Sam*, was murdered by a nineteen-year-old Tucson man named Robert John Bardo. Bardo had been obsessed with Schaeffer ever since she sent him an autographed photograph in response to his fan letter. He built a shrine in his room out of other photos of her and videotapes of her shows.

When Bardo saw Schaeffer acting out a bedroom scene in a movie, he decided that she had to be killed for her "immorality." He went to California to seek her out. He found out where she lived, hid outside her apartment, and shot her in cold blood as she stood helplessly in her doorway. Bardo was arrested, convicted, and sentenced to life in prison.

Madonna was also the victim of an erotomaniac. In 1995 the Material Girl was hounded by a homeless man named

Robert Hoskins, who believed that she was his wife. When she ignored him, he threatened to cut her throat. Hoskins was eventually arrested, convicted, and sentenced to prison.

Erotomania is a favorite subject of literature and of films such as *Fatal Attraction* and *American Beauty*. Some people have suggested that when John Hinckley shot President Ronald Reagan, he was partially motivated by his own erotomania as well as the related erotomania theme in the film *Taxi Driver*. In the film, the creepy taxi-driver character played by Robert De Niro becomes obsessed with rescuing the twelve-year-old prostitute character played by Jodie Foster. In real life, John Hinckley declared after the shooting incident, "I did it for Jodie."

DOCTORS, DOCTORS, AND MORE DOCTORS

Wendy Scott learned early in life that being sick could get her a lot of attention. As an adult, she managed to get herself admitted to over six hundred hospitals over the course of twelve years. During that time she convinced doctors to perform forty-two unnecessary surgeries on her.

Her illness? She suffered from Munchausen syndrome.

Munchausen syndrome is a rare disorder in which a person goes from doctor to doctor, and from hospital to hospital, seeking treatment for symptoms that do not exist. We're not talking garden-variety hypochondria ("I have a weird headache; omigod, maybe it's a tumor!"); we're talking about someone who makes a career out of lying to medical personnel in order to be admitted, poked, prodded, and even operated on repeatedly—all for the sake of being a permanent patient and getting attention. Once admitted to the hospital, the Munchausen patient often quarrels with doctors and nurses in order to get even *more* attention.

Some Munchausen cases involve feigning illness; for example, a person might collapse outside a hospital, pretending to have a heart attack, or complain of severe abdominal pains in order to convince the doctors to perform exploratory surgery. In Katherine Ramsland's CourtTV article "Factitious Disorders," she describes a case—chronicled by Charles Ford in his book *Lies! Lies! Lies! The Psychology of Deceit*—about a man who on several occasions faked renal failure on airplanes and caused emergency landings.

Still other cases have a masochistic component; for example, a person might induce vomiting by various means, perform self-mutilation, or swallow inappropriate substances or objects (including, by some accounts, dinner forks) in order to get medical attention. Some Munchausen patients will inject themselves with fecal matter to produce symptoms. In an anonymous posting on a Munchausen Web site, one woman wrote that as a teen she burned her arms with oven cleaner and put kitchen cleansers in her juice. Her bladder eventually had to be removed as a result of the damage she had done to her system. She also admitted to inducing frostbite and injecting bacteria into her bloodstream.

Also known as hospital addiction, hospital hobo, permanent patient, and Van Gogh's syndrome (after the artist who cut off his own ear), Munchausen syndrome was named by medical writer Richard Asher in 1951. Baron Munchausen is a fictitious character created by the novelist Rudolf Eric Raspe, based on the real-life Karl Friedrich Hieronymus von Münch-hausen of Hanover, who was famous for telling outrageously improbable tall tales.

Obviously, Munchausen syndrome can be financially and otherwise draining on the health care system. According to the Web site www.whonamedit.com, the 1993 *Guinness Book of World Records* cites a Munchausen patient named William McIloy who cost Britain's National Health Service approximately $4 million over fifty years. McIloy underwent four hundred presumably unnecessary operations in a hundred different hospitals using twenty-two separate aliases.

There are several variations on the Munchausen theme. With Munchausen's mammae syndrome, a woman with normal, healthy breasts will request an excessive number of breast exams, mammograms, and so forth. (No comment.)

In his article "Munchausen by Internet: Faking Illness Online," Marc D. Feldman describes the apparent phenomenon of Munchausen patients seeking attention not from doctors but from online support groups. These patients will click from one support group to another, pretending to have whatever illness or condition is particular to each group. Some will even use different aliases to assume multiple identities within one group—for example, the patient, the patient's worried parent, and the patient's worried spouse—in order to create a believable and urgent scenario of illness and ensuing family crisis. Feldman coined the terms *Munchausen by Internet* and *Virtual Factitious Disorder* to describe this variation.

The most disturbing Munchausen variation of all may be Munchausen syndrome by proxy. With this illness, a parent, usually the mother, will invent symptoms in her own child, causing the child to be subjected to unnecessary and often uncomfortable or painful examinations and treatments. In the "active" form of this syndrome, the parent will inflict harm on the child—suffocating the child for a few minutes, injecting the child with insulin in order to induce a hypoglycemic coma, etc.—in order to create real symptoms. In the "passive" form, the parent will merely fabricate the symptoms on behalf of the child, or somehow teach the child to complain about fictitious symptoms on his or her own. This syndrome is a form of battered-child syndrome and is considered to be a peculiar—and horrifying—type of child abuse.

GILLE DE LA TOURETTE'S SYNDROME

As a child, the man suffered from constant throat clearing and nervous coughing. As an adult he developed vocal tics as well, and found himself emitting short, random noises at inopportune moments. His motor tics grew to include certain twitching, smelling, and hitting behaviors that seemed to relieve his inner tension, his ever-present psychological "itch."

This description is typical of someone with Gille de la Tourette's syndrome. Often referred to simply as Tourette's, Gille de la Tourette's syndrome is a rare neurological disorder characterized by echolalia (automatically repeating others' utterances), palilalia (automatically repeating one's own utterances), coprolalia (compulsively saying dirty words), and echopraxia (involuntarily mimicking the movements of others, lack of muscular coordination, and facial and bodily spasms). Not surprisingly, people with Gille de la Tourette's syndrome find it hard to fit in socially or to concentrate on tasks.

The onset of this disease is often in childhood, from the ages of 2 to 15, but it can appear later. It affects three times as many boys as girls. Teenagers with Gille de la Tourette's syndrome can be disturbingly free and loose with the obscenities, whereas adults will often try to mask such outbursts with coughing. Affected teens can also experience sleep disturbances and self-mutilation.

Some experts suspect that the British writer Dr. Samuel Johnson suffered from Gille de la Tourette's syndrome. Others suspect that Wolfgang Amadeus Mozart, who had a penchant for dirty talk and nonsense words, had the syndrome as well.

DOWN THE RABBIT HOLE

You slip down into a rabbit hole and find that everyone and everything around you is unnaturally small. Time passes so, *so* slowly. No, you're not on hallucinogenic drugs. You may, however, be suffering from Alice-in-Wonderland syndrome.

Named in 1955 by an English psychiatrist, John Todd, after Lewis Carroll's fictional character, this psychiatric syndrome causes its victim to experience distortions of space, time, and body image. People look tiny and Lilliputian; in fact, this syndrome is also called Lilliputian syndrome, after Jonathan Swift's *Gulliver's Travels*, in which the intrepid Gulliver encounters wee little people in the land of Lilliput.

Other symptoms of this mysterious syndrome include feelings of levitation, dreamlike or trancelike states, delirium, and a distorted sense of one's own body image. One Alice-in-Wonderland patient reported feeling a "Tweedle-dee, Tweedle-dum" sensation: She felt bizarrely and uncharacteristically short and wide as she walked along.

One theory behind Lewis Carroll's creation of Alice's character is that he suffered severely from migraines and might have experienced Alice's sensations down the rabbit hole as a result of his headaches. Alice-in-Wonderland syndrome has been linked to migraines; in fact, a majority of patients have a personal or family history of them.

Incidentally, another medical term was derived from *Alice's Adventures in Wonderland*: Cheshire cat syndrome, first described in 1968 by the British physician Eric George Lapthorne Bywaters, according to the Who Named It? Web site (www.whonamedit.com).

MORBID JEALOUSY

Speaking of mental illnesses named after literary characters (and speaking of mental illnesses named after literary characters by the English psychiatrist John Todd), there's Othello, that unhappy Moor of Venice. In Shakespeare's play, Othello suspects, wrongfully, that his loving wife, Desdemona, is cheating on him. Deaf to her pleas and entreaties, he strangles her to death in a fit of jealousy.

Many centuries later we have Othello syndrome, more commonly known as "delusional jealousy." Those who suffer from this disorder are morbidly and psychotically jealous, often for no good reason. The manifestation of their jealousy can range from verbal threats to murder.

KLEPTOMANIA

Kleptomania is a rare disorder whose principal symptom is compulsive stealing. Many shoplifters are referred to casually as "kleptos," but true kleptomania is a much less common illness than many people think. It is also much more complicated than, for example, a teenager's occasional dark urge to lift CDs or cosmetics.

Kleptomaniacs steal repeatedly, and they steal things they don't particularly need or want. The lifted items are often returned, replaced, hidden, or thrown away altogether. The act of stealing evokes a range of strong emotional responses in kleptomaniacs: tension before and during the act, then elation upon the successful completion of the act, followed by major guilt and fear of discovery.

Kleptomaniacs tend to suffer from the eating disorder anorexia nervosa and/or depression. The cause of this disorder is as yet unknown. Most kleptomaniacs do not seek treatment unless they have been arrested and are ordered to do so by the courts.

THE WOLF WOMAN

In their *American Journal of Psychiatry* article "A Case of Lycanthropy," as excerpted in the Primitivism Web site, Drs. Harvey

Rostentock and Kenneth R. Vincent describe the strange case of a forty-nine-year-old woman who believed herself to be a wolf.

According to the article, the woman felt "like an animal with claws." A married woman, she was consumed with day-dreams about sex with other women and with animals.

Things reached a critical point at a family get-together when the woman stripped, assumed an on-all-fours position, and "offered herself to her mother." The next night, after having sex with her husband, she "growled, scratched, and gnawed at the bed" for two hours.

The woman was admitted for inpatient treatment. Despite medication and psychotherapy, she continued to act in a wolf-like manner. According to Rostenstock and Vincent's article, she was taken to ranting such statements as: "I am a wolf of the night; I am wolf woman of the day. . . . I have claws, teeth, fangs, hair . . . and anguish is my prey at night . . . the gnashing and snarling of teeth . . . powerless is my cause, I am what I am and will always roam the earth after death. . . . I will continue to search for perfection and salvation." As she ranted, she was overcome by sexual excitement as well as the urge to kill.

When the woman gazed in the mirror, she saw a wolf's head and not her own face. She made incoherent animal grunts constantly. Her doctors saw some improvement over time, although she had a brief relapse one night when there was a full moon.

This is a classic case of lycanthropy, a rare disorder in which people believe themselves to be werewolves. There are many other modern-day cases of lycanthropy in the literature. The Web site article "Modern Werewolf Cases from Scientific Viewpoints" describes several interesting cases taken from a 1975 issue of the *The Canadian Journal of Psychiatry*. In one, a 20-

year-old man believed that he was sprouting fur on his hands and face; he was also obsessed with chasing, catching, and chowing down on live rabbits. In another case, a 37-year-old man howled at the moon and slept in cemeteries.

The legend—or reality, according to some—of the werewolf has been around for many centuries. Werewolves were beings that appeared to be human and could transform themselves into wolves or into half-wolf, half-human creatures. They could do this at will, except at the full moon, when the transformation occurred involuntarily.

According to David Sheldon in his Web site article "The Legend of the Werewolf," lycanthropy was a recognized illness in the Middle Ages. It was believed then that lycanthropes *thought* they could turn themselves into werewolves but did not actually do so, or that they could run around acting like werewolves and even engage in murder and cannibalism.

The difference between then and now (for the most part) is that back then, people really believed that *true* werewolves also existed, in addition to lycanthropes.

Werewolves were much feared in the Middle Ages. Consequently, people suspected of being werewolves were constantly hunted by those who wanted to clear the land of their scourge. Citizens of that time believed it was possible to tell a werewolf while it was in its human form. Such wolf people were very hairy, and even had hair sprouting from their palms. They had small, pointy ears and one continuous, bushy eyebrow. The third finger of each hand was as long as the second. Men who fitted this description were always closely watched.

According to Sheldon, a werewolf was thought to be able to turn his skin inside out in order to hide his fur while he was in his

"human" state. This led to the rather horrific practice of peasants ripping open people's bodies in search of werewolf fur.

In later centuries it was thought that a werewolf could be
killed only with a bullet made of silver or from a melted-down
crucifix, or by a knife whose blade was made of such metal.
The dead werewolf then had to be burned: Merely burying it
would enable it to return as a vampire. (No doubt a very *angry*
vampire.)

There were various explanations as to how one became a
werewolf to begin with. Sheldon's article contains some colorful examples. A Russian legend said that one could become a
werewolf by jumping over a fallen tree in a forest, stabbing the
tree with a copper knife, and chanting a spell. Other ways
included finding an animal that had been killed by a wolf and
eating its brains, and drinking water that had pooled in a
wolf's paw print.

According to Sheldon, a more elaborate method was to
make an ointment that included, among other things, wolfs-
bane, foxglove, opium, bat blood, and the fat of a child who
had been murdered. Then the would-be werewolf was to rub
the ointment all over himself and don a wolfskin pelt. This
would ensure that he would morph into a wolf every night.

The history books note a boy named Jean Grenier who
lived in France in the seventeenth century. He was fond of eating raw human flesh. Over the course of several years he ate
over fifty children, including a crying baby whom he dragged
out of its house. After attacking a local girl (who survived),
Jean Grenier was arrested and tried by the parliament of Bor-
deaux. The girl claimed that she had been jumped by a furry
red beast while she was minding the sheep. Witnesses backed

up the girl with their accounts of other, similar attacks.

Two doctors testified that Jean Grenier suffered from lycanthropy. The judge didn't buy the lycanthropy explanation and sentenced Grenier to life imprisonment in a monastery, where he was often seen moving about on all fours and consuming whatever raw meat he could get his hands (or paws) on.

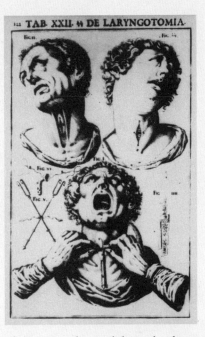

According to Sheldon, there are tales and legends about other types of were-creatures around the world: werecats in Germany; werefoxes in Japan and China; wereboars in Scandinavia; and werehares in Wales—in other words, witches that turned themselves into hares and sucked the milk out of cows.

Modern-day experts speculate that rabies may provide an explanation for some of the lycanthropic behavior displayed in the Middle Ages. Foaming at the mouth and the furious urge to bite are two of the symptoms of rabies. A wolf displaying such symptoms could with a bite have passed them along to a human, who would then feel and appear "wolflike" to himself and others.

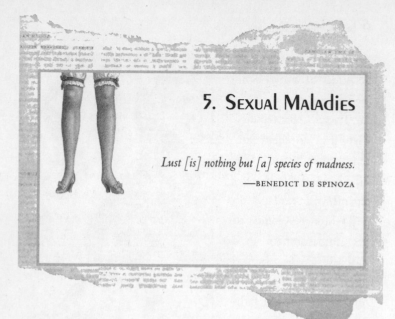

5. Sexual Maladies

Lust [is] nothing but [a] species of madness.
—BENEDICT DE SPINOZA

SEX IS A WONDERFUL, BIZARRE, AND INTENSELY PERsonal thing. What people do behind closed doors in order to give themselves and their partners pleasure can (and should) range from the routine to the sublime, from five minutes of the missionary position to sky's-the-limit kinkiness.

Unfortunately, there are many factors that can get in the way of a satisfying sex life, including relationship problems, no relationship at all, feelings of shame and guilt, lack of experience, illness, hormonal imbalances, and alcohol or drug abuse. The list goes on. There are also many common conditions that can inhibit pleasure: impotence, premature ejaculation, and pain during intercourse, to name just a few.

There can be serious anatomical problems as well. For example, Peyronie's disease can in severe cases cause the penis to bend during erection, making intercourse uncomfortable and unwieldy. With a condition known as ambiguous genitalia, a person is born with genitals that don't read precisely "male" or "female." For example, a male may have a penis so small that it resembles a large clitoris. Likewise, a female may have a clitoris so large that it resembles a penis, or an oddly shaped labium that resembles a scrotum.

In this chapter, you will read about sexual maladies that one doesn't often hear about. As you will see, the behaviors associated with them fall somewhere in the gray area between normal and abnormal (although many may seem squarely on the extreme end of abnormal). Some of them have to do with an inability to have sex except under very extreme conditions. Some have to do with an inability to have sex without exhibiting peculiar symptoms. Many of these disorders have a physical or psychological basis, although some remain a complete enigma to the experts.

Also sprinkled throughout the chapter are little tidbits and trivia about what people do in the privacy of their bedrooms (and elsewhere), many of them gleaned from the information-rich Internet.

SEX REMEDIES

Men and women have used aphrodisiacs throughout history to stimulate their sexual appetites. Named after the Greek goddess of love, Aphrodite, aphrodisiacs can come in many forms, including beverages, foods, drugs, and scents.

We've all heard about popular aphrodisiacs such as chocolates and oysters. According to the Improving Sex Web site (www.improvingsex.com), oysters are thought to be passion-provoking because they contain zinc, which can rev up vaginal lubrication as well as sperm and testosterone production. There is a legend that Casanova ate fifty oysters every morning in his bath with his lover. Hindu lovemaking manuals and other historical sources also mention onions as an effective aphrodisiac.

A number of spices and herbs are thought to have sexy properties. Cardamom is used in India as a cure for premature ejaculation and impotence. The Greeks, Romans, Egyptians, Japanese, and Chinese have a long history of imbibing garlic as an aphrodisiac. Cloves, vanilla, and saffron are also reputed to be highly stimulating.

An article on aphrodisiacs on www.thesite.org mentions some exotic (and, frankly, really weird) love potions. Some of them date back thousands of years. Some of them are highly illegal. They include jackal bile, snake blood, deer testicles, tiger bones, rhino horns, and the penises of seals or deer.

One well-known aphrodisiac, "Spanish fly," is actually the crushed carcass of the dried emerald-green blister beetle. According to the Improving Sex Web site, legend has it that the Roman empress Livia used to slip Spanish fly into the foods and beverages of people she wished to blackmail; she figured that the drug would drive them to do all sorts of compromising things. In the eighteenth century the Marquis de Sade gave it to prostitutes in the hope of getting a really fun party going.

Unfortunately, Spanish fly is very poisonous and can lead to serious illness and even death. In the Marquis de Sade's case, the poor prostitutes became sick, and the marquis was arrested and tried for poisoning.

The Improving Sex Web site mentions another aphrodisiac with nasty side effects: *chan su*, a drug made from the skin of toads. It has been sold in the U.S. under the names "Rock Hard" and "Stone." *Chan su* has its roots in China, where it was originally used as a topical anesthetic. People began ingesting it as an aphrodisiac when it was found to possess potency-increasing properties. However, *chan su* contains cardiac steroids that can lead to heart problems and even death.

Another aphrodisiac listed on the Improving Sex Web site is *yohimbe*, an herb that comes from a West African tree *(Corynanthe yohimbe)*. West Africans swear by it. Veterinarians have used it to cure impotence in stallions.

Then, of course, there is Viagra. Produced by Pfizer and approved by the FDA in 1998, Viagra is the brand name of sildenafil citrate. The now-famous little blue pill helps men achieve and maintain an erection, in some cases for a very, very, *very* long time. Viagra's appeal is not limited to men. Women have jumped on the Viagra bandwagon as well, despite FDA warnings against women and children using this drug.

And last but not least, let's not forget those green M&M's.

UNUSUAL REACTIONS TO SEX

People have been known to display very curious reactions to sex. According to Robert M. Youngson's book *Medical Curiosities,* there are recorded cases of people who break into hiccups or start vomiting during the act. Youngson's book also refers to a *St. Louis Medical Journal* report about a man who began sneezing every time sex was even contemplated, and another report, in the *The New England Journal of Medicine,* about a man who went blind in one eye right before orgasm. The blindness would last for a few minutes, then his vision would be restored.

Perhaps the most dramatic case in Youngson's book is about a man who lost all sensation in his member at the moment of orgasm. Even worse, the numbness was replaced by excruciating pain if he tried to withdraw or even make the slightest move- ment. It was necessary for him to remain very still just where he was, until his penis grew totally flaccid. This could sometimes take up to an hour, causing him and his wife much discomfort.

PRIAPISM

Imagine one's penis being erect for many hours without one's feeling any sexual arousal whatsoever. The penis is clogged with blood, and there is lots of pain involved. This condition, known as priapism, occurs when blood cannot drain from the penis. An underlying disorder can be the cause, such as leuke- mia, sickle-cell anemia, or various nervous system diseases.

Priapism is named after the Greek god Priapos, who sym- bolizes fertility and sexuality and is often depicted in statues and other artwork as a guy with a very big, very tumescent appendage. Priapism is not a means to cheap out on Viagra but a dangerous condition requiring immediate medical attention. Treatment usually involves surgery and draining of the blood.

DO I EAT IT OR DO I HAVE SEX WITH IT?

It is common practice for people to masturbate with the assistance of common or not-so-common objects. The casebooks and sex manuals list vacuum cleaners, bottles, and even bayonet tubes and bathtub faucets, just to name a few examples.

Kluver-Bucy syndrome is another kettle of fish altogether. Symptoms of this rare and mysterious condition can include oral confusion and hypersexuality or indiscriminate sexuality. According to a Web site article called "A Collection of Unusual Neurological States," one man suffering from this illness was arrested while trying to have sex with the pavement.

With this disorder, a person may try to put some inappropriate object in his or her mouth or attempt to have sex with it. According to an article on the Library of Neuropsychological Information Web site, this condition was first observed in monkeys and is believed to be the result of neurological damage to the front of the temporal lobe and the amygdala, a portion of the brain that is part of the limbic system. Some describe people (and monkeys) suffering from this disorder as not being able to tell the difference between food, a sexual mate, prey, and objects in general.

THE CASE OF THE MISSING PENIS

A Nigerian woman was almost lynched by a crowd because a market trader accused her of stealing his penis.

Did she really steal his penis? No. The man was suffering from a delusional psychopathology known as koro. With koro, a man believes that his genitals have been stolen or that they are shrinking into his body for good.

According to a Web site article called "Koro: A Natural History of Penis Panic" by a person named Vaughan (just Vaughan), koro has been observed for thousands of years and in different cultures all over the world. One of the first documented cases of koro was mentioned around 300 B.C., in a Chinese medical text known as *The Yellow Emperor's Classic of Internal Medicine*.

Vaughan cites many cases of actual koro "epidemics." In Singapore in 1967, hospitals were besieged with men who were panic-stricken about their supposedly shrinking penises. Some of them had even tried to keep their penises from shrinking with clamps and other means. This particular koro outbreak may have been caused by rumors that there was bad pork on the market that could potentially cause genital shrinkage.

Koro "epidemics" were also reported in the 1980s in the Guangdong province of China, where men apparently went into penis panic when they sighted a beautiful fox spirit who was known to rob men of their genitals.

According to Vaughan's article, in Africa koro may or may not be related to beliefs about sorcerers and black magic. Sometimes a man will accuse a stranger who has touched him of stealing his penis. In a 1990 koro outbreak in Nigeria, some of the men who believed that their penises had been stolen from them also believed that their penises were eventually returned. They would even go so far as to disrobe in public to demonstrate that fact, although a man would occasionally claim that he had been given back the wrong penis—a vastly shrunken one.

Koro has been related to bad marijuana, brain tumors, stroke, schizophrenia, and depression as well as cultural and social factors.

BESTIALITY

For some, human beings are not the sexual partners of choice. Indeed, there are those who prefer carnal experiences with pets such as dogs and cats or even farm animals such as cows, sheep, chickens, and horses.

There are even more unusual examples of sex with animals. According to the World Sex Records Web site, in ancient Rome, women were reputed to have pleasured themselves with the heads of live snakes. There are tales of live fish being used to similar effect.

Though many individuals and cultures may condemn the practice of sex with animals, others are more tolerant of this practice. The World Sex Records Web site contains several examples. The Copper Eskimos, who inhabited the Arctic coast of North America, were known to practice intercourse with animals, alive or dead. The Masai people of Kenya and Hopi Indians were also said to have practiced bestiality. This Web site mentions a Fez legend—"Fez" probably referring to the city in Morocco—of a man who used magic to deflower seventy-two virgin cows in one night. Fishermen of certain parts of the East

African coast are reputed to have intercourse with dead female dugongs (large aquatic mammals) that they have killed. This act is apparently necessary in order to chase away the ghosts of the dead dugongs so that they don't pursue their hunters.

The World Sex Records Web site also mentions "animal prostitutes" throughout history. In certain "ancient temples" of unspecified geography and religion, baboons, monkeys, and other types of animals were taught to engage in coitus with both men and women; the priests stood by and accepted payment for the animals' services. Dogs, goats, geese, and turkeys have also been popular animal prostitutes. The Web site adds that today in some parts of the world, there are live interspecies sex shows where audiences pay money to watch women copulating with horses and other four-legged friends.

Bestiality is considered by some to be a type of paraphilia (see below).

PARAPHILIAS

Paraphilia is an umbrella term for a number of sexual deviations. The *DSM-IV* (*Diagnostic and Statistical Manual of Mental Disorders*, fourth edition) defines paraphilias as "being characterized by recurrent, intense sexual fantasies, urges, or behaviors that involve unusual objects, activities, or situations and cause clinically significant distress or impairment in social, occupational, or other important areas of functioning." These fantasies, urges, or behaviors can involve inanimate objects, suffering (real or imagined), humiliation (of one's partner or oneself), and sometimes nonconsenting partners.

Paraphilias can be problematic for a number of reasons. For one thing, they can be seriously debilitating to one's professional and personal lives. For example, people who suffer from a major shoe fetish are going to have a hard time forming relationships with anyone or anything other than shoes. Also, those who suffer from paraphilias are often unable to perform sexually or experience sexual pleasure without the necessary fantasies and behaviors, whether we're talking shoes, bondage equipment, or partners dressed as prison wardens. The behavior tends to be obsessive.

Still, some of the behaviors involved in paraphilias may, in the context of a healthy sexual relationship (with oneself or with a partner), be considered "normal" experimentation, whatever *normal* means in the universe of sexuality. Sex can, and should, push the limits. It's only when the limits are pushed too far that paraphiles' behavior can raise eyebrows (as well as psychiatric red flags).

According to the Discovery.com health Web site, paraphilias are more common in men than women. Many of the paraphilias are rare. The most common paraphilias include pedophilia, voyeurism, and exhibitionism.

There are also a number of not-so-common paraphilias. The following entries are examples of the latter, many of them gleaned from the highly enlightening Dictionary of Sexuality Web site.

APOTEMNOPHILIA

With apotemnophilia, sexual arousal and pleasure are dependent on, and responsive to, being an amputee. (A variation on apotemnophilia is acrotomophilia, in which one fantasizes that his or her lover is an amputee.) An apotemnophile can become sexually obsessed with getting a limb amputated, either by someone else or via self-amputation. Some people with this paraphilia will strap on household appliances in order to simulate the sensation of wearing prosthetics.

According to a December 6, 1998, article in South Africa's *Sunday Times*, a 70-something unlicensed surgeon in California and an 80-year-old man had a relationship based on apotemnophilia. The man had paid the surgeon $10,000 to remove a healthy leg. The operation went wrong, and the man died a few days later from gangrene. The surgeon was arrested and charged with causing the man's death.

ASPHYXIOPHILIA

With asphyxiophilia, sexual arousal and pleasure are dependent on, and responsive to, asphyxiation, but not to the point of loss of consciousness. This can be done by hanging or strangulation, or by the use of plastic bags or gags. Needless to say, split-second timing is essential, especially when the practice is autoerotic. Many cases have resulted in accidental death.

One asphyxiophile described his habits on the Sexuality.org Web site by writing, "My goal is to get off and escape without passing out and dying."

CHRONOPHILIA

Chronophilia is an umbrella term for paraphilias in which sexual arousal and pleasure are dependent on, and responsive to, impersonating an older or younger person in relation to one's sexual partner. Examples include infantilism, ephebophilia (aka Lolita syndrome), and gerontalism, or gerontophilia, in which one's sexual partner must be parental or grandparental in age.

With one kind of chronophilia called autonepiophilia, sexual arousal and pleasure are dependent on, and responsive to, pretending to be a baby in diapers and having one's sexual partner play along. This practice can be accompanied by discipline and humiliation rituals.

COPROPHILIA

With coprophilia, sexual arousal and pleasure are dependent on, and responsive to, activities involving feces. This can involve enemas, defecation, and various forms of fecal play: smelling, smearing, eating, etc. *Scat* is the vernacular term for this practice, from the Greek term *skatos*, meaning dung. The term *klismaphilia* specifically refers to sexual pleasure and excitement from giving and receiving enemas.

EMETOPHILIA

With emetophilia, sexual arousal and pleasure are dependent on, and responsive to, vomiting during sex, being vomited on, inducing oneself to vomit, or inducing one's partner to vomit. The vomit can be directed onto one's body or, in some cases, into one's body, for example, into the mouth. This behavior can be part of an S and M dynamic.

There are various Web sites for emetophiles, including Vomit Online (www.vomitonline.com). Vomit Online's stated goals are to "provide content in a number of forms," including "puke alert[s] regarding vomit scenes on TV (reality-based not fake vomit)" and "our original vomit video series 'The Emeto-Files.'"

FORMICOPHILIA

With formicophilia, sexual arousal and pleasure are dependent on, and responsive to, the use of insects during sex. One practice involves spreading honey, jam, or another sweet, sticky substance on the genitals and waiting for flies, ants, or other bugs to land and titillate. Some formicophiles enjoy inserting insects into their vaginas or rectums and feeling the sensation of the critters trying to escape.

With a practice known as "crush fetishism," a person becomes sexually aroused by crushing insects or watching another person crush insects, such as a woman grinding a bug under her heel. According to Professor G. A. Pearson's article "Insect Fetish Objects," there is an international community

of "crush freaks" who sub-
scribe to such magazines
as the *American Journal of the
Crush Freaks* and *Squish!*

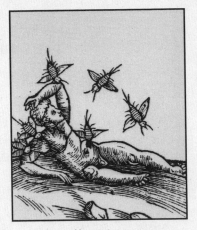

Professor Pearson's ar-
ticle also describes several
videotape titles for crush
fetishists, including *Squish
Playhouse #3* ("starring Deb-
bie the Crush Queen and
costarring dozens of crick-
ets and mealworms") and *Squish Playhouse #5* ("featuring a special guest victim—a tarantula spider!"). The article mentions
the popularity of audiotapes as well, including *A Housewife's
Guide to Squishing Bugs* ("Follow her from kitchen to garden as
she steps on her victims with no mercy!").

NECROPHILIA

Necrophilia is a sexual attraction to the dead. There are
some interesting historical examples of necrophilia mentioned
on the Armageddon Entertainment Web site. The ancient
Egyptians commonly did not have corpses embalmed for a few
days, so that those inclined to necrophilia could enjoy the
bodies first. Herod allegedly slept next to his dead wife Mari-
anne for seven years. The emperor Charlemagne likewise refused to let go of the remains of his German paramour, and
Queen Juana of Castile kept her dead husband, Philip the
Handsome, close by for three years.

PARAPHILIAS

ABASIOPHILIA

With abasiophilia, sexual arousal and pleasure are dependent on, and responsive to, a lame or crippled sexual partner. It is common for abasiophiles to be obsessed with people who wear orthopedic leg braces, such as those associated with polio, spina bifida, and cerebral palsy.

AGALMATOPHILIA

With agalmatophilia, one is sexually attracted to a nude statue or mannequin. There can also be a sadistic component whereby the person gets off on mutilating a statue or mannequin while masturbating. This paraphilia is also called statuophilia and pygmalionism.

AUTAGONISTOPHILIA

With autagonistophilia, sexual arousal and pleasure are dependent on, and responsive to, being watched, being on camera, or being onstage.

AUTOASSASSINOPHILIA

With autoassassinophilia, sexual arousal and pleasure are dependent on, and responsive to, staging the possibility of one's own assassination at another's hand.

CATHETEROPHILIA

With catheterophilia, sexual arousal and pleasure are dependent on, and responsive to, having a catheter inserted into the urethra.

CHREMATISTOPHILIA

With chrematistophilia, sexual arousal and pleasure are dependent on, and responsive to, being forced to pay for sex. Another turn-on is actually being robbed by the sexual partner.

ELECTROCUTOPHILIA

With electrocutophilia, sexual arousal and pleasure are dependent on, and responsive to, electrically stimulating the anal-rectal area, penis, scrotum, vagina, clitoris, vulva, urethra, nipples, and other choice body parts. This can be part of an S and M ritual. Unfortunately, accidental death can occur if one is not careful.

KLEPTOPHILIA

With kleptophilia, sexual arousal and pleasure are dependent on, and responsive to, illegally entering and stealing stuff from the home of a potential sexual partner, who may or may not be a stranger. This behavior may or may not involve forcefully demanding sex.

MYSOPHILIA

With mysophilia, sexual arousal and pleasure are dependent on, and responsive to, smelling, tasting, chewing, or otherwise getting off on sweaty underwear, soiled clothing, and tampons or menstrual pads (presumably used). Self-degradation and self-humiliation play a large role in this behavior.

NASOPHILIA

With nasophilia, sexual arousal and pleasure are dependent on, and responsive to, touching, sucking, licking, or simply looking at a person's nose.

(cont.)

SCOPTOPHILIA

With scoptophilia, sexual arousal and pleasure are dependent on, and responsive to, watching other people have sex. This is different from voyeurism in that the watching is not done surreptitiously but openly and by arrangement.

SIDERODROMOPHILIA

With siderodromophilia, sexual arousal and pleasure are dependent on, and responsive to, riding on trains.

SOMNOPHILIA

Also known as the "sleeping princess syndrome," this paraphilia involves sexual arousal and pleasure being dependent on, and responsive to, sneaking up on a sleeping stranger and waking the person with kisses, caresses, oral sex, etc. Somnophilia does not involve violence or force.

SYMPHOROPHILIA

With symphorophilia, sexual arousal and pleasure are dependent on, and responsive to, staging the possibility of, or waiting for, a traffic accident or other disaster.

TAPHEPHILIA

With taphephilia, sexual arousal and pleasure are dependent on, and responsive to, being buried alive.

UROPHILIA

With urophilia, sexual arousal and pleasure are dependent on, and responsive to, being urinated on or urinating on someone (aka "golden showers"), watching someone urinate, and so forth. This practice is often referred to as "water sports." The term *renifleurism* refers to being sexually attracted to the smell of urine.

A MISCELLANY OF UNUSUAL
SEXUAL TERMS

The following is an assortment of sex-related words and phrases that one doesn't often come across in everyday conversation:

- **Astringent treatment.** The use of chemicals to shrink the mucous membranes of the vagina, usually for the purposes of simulating a state of virginity.
- **Avisodomy.** Sex with a bird. According to the World Sex Records Web site, the Marquis de Sade wrote that turkeys were commonly used in Parisian whorehouses for sexual purposes. Not for the faint-of-heart, one method of enhancing orgasm in these situations was for the man to behead the poor turkey at the moment of ejaculation; the bird's sudden rise in body temperature and final death spasms were believed to heighten the experience.
- **Axillary intercourse.** The use of a person's armpit for sex, e.g., when a man thrusts his penis into his partner's armpit.
- **Frotteurism.** Rubbing one's body against other people without their permission for purposes of sexual excitement.
- **Oculolinctus.** Licking someone's eyeball for sexual pleasure.

- **Partialism.** Being sexually attracted to a certain part of a person's body without being sexually attracted to the person as a whole.
- **Telephone scatologia.** The obsessive urge to make obscene phone calls.

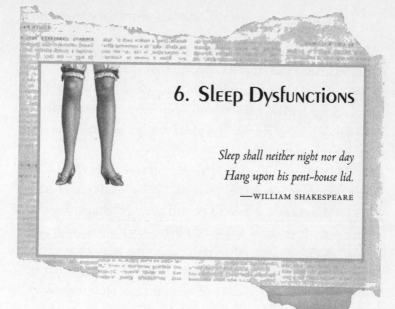

6. Sleep Dysfunctions

Sleep shall neither night nor day
Hang upon his pent-house lid.
—WILLIAM SHAKESPEARE

Most of us know what it is like to have sleepless nights—those endless dark stretches of tossing and turning, staring at the clock, stressing out about deadlines, counting sheep, and cursing that extra cup of coffee we absolutely should not have had.

However, there are a number of sleep problems that involve more complicated symptoms than, say, occasional bouts of insomnia or waking up groggy and cranky once in a while. Unfortunately, these problems are far more common than we might think.

Sleep is a complex process involving five distinct stages: Stage I, light sleep; stages 2, 3, and 4, deep sleep; and REM (rapid eye movement) sleep. If all goes well, we cycle through these stages several times each night in this order: I-2-3-4-3-2-REM-2-3-4-3-2-REM, and so on, until we wake up in the morning.

The more REM stages we experience, the more rested we will feel in the morning. Interruption to the cycle will result in fewer of these restorative REM "hits," since we have to start from Stage 1 all over again. Such interruptions can come from crying infants, neighbors who play Pearl Jam at three A.M., and other external sources.

They can also happen as a result of sleep disorders. One fairly common sleep disorder is restless leg syndrome (RLS). RLS sufferers find it hard to lie still during the night because their legs drive them absolutely berserk: aches, itching, tingling, prickling, and other really annoying sensations. They feel the urge to move their legs around—flexing, bending, stretching, whatever it takes to make the discomfort go away. Sometimes the only relief is to get up in the middle of the night and walk around the house like the ghost of Hamlet's father, or to take a hot shower. Unfortunately, the discomfort often returns as soon as the person goes back to bed.

And as if one strange leg-related sleep disorder weren't enough, many people with RLS also have period limb movement syndrome, or PLMS. Unlike RLS, the PLMS symptoms manifest themselves while the person is actually asleep. The primary symptom is a periodic jerking of the legs that cause minor, brief sleep interruptions that the person may or may not be aware of. Although PLMS may not cause discomfort to the sleeper in the way that RLS does, it can cause much sleepiness and yawning during the daytime.

Another common sleep disorder is bruxism, or grinding the teeth during sleep. Also referred to as nocturnal bruxism, nocturnal tooth grinding, and nocturnal tooth clenching, this condition can do a number on one's teeth over time (imagine the nightly wear and tear), annoy sleepmates (imagine finger-nails on a chalkboard times ten), and lead to jaw discomfort and damage.

But these three sleep disorders, while troubling, can be relatively benign compared to some of the more serious ones, known as parasomnias. Similar to *paraphilia, parasomnia* is a catchall term for a group of related sleep disorders. Parasom-nias are characterized by peculiar, unsleeplike behavior during sleep. Some stranger examples of things parasomniacs have done while asleep include cleaning the house, moving and rearranging furniture, and cooking and consuming an entire meal. Some parasomniacs have reportedly tried to eat ciga-rettes and raw bacon in their sleep. Parasomniacs do not re-member their nighttime shenanigans the next day. If there are no "witnesses" to their behavior, their only clues to their para-somnia might be food stains on their pillow or a mysteriously redecorated room.

The following are several examples of sleep disorders that fall into the "parasomnia" category: sleepwalking (or som-nambulism), sleep-related eating disorder, sleep talking, sleep terrors, REM movement disorder, and multiple sleep disorder —as well as an additional one which some experts consider to be a new parasomnia: "sexual behaviors during sleep."

SLEEPWALKING

In 1981, a Scottsdale, Arizona, man named Steven Steinberg was accused of fatally stabbing his wife twenty-six times with a kitchen knife. According to an article titled "Can Sleepwalking

Be a Murder Defense?" by Dr. Lawrence Martin, Steinberg admitted to the murder, but claimed he committed the heinous deed while sleepwalking and therefore could not be considered sane at the time. A psychiatrist testified that Steinberg was in a state of "dissociative reaction" during the attack. The jury agreed and acquitted Steinberg for reasons of temporary insanity.

Dr. Martin also wrote about Kenneth Parks, a twenty-three-year-old Toronto man who got up one morning in 1987, got into his car, drove to his in-laws', stabbed his mother-in-law to death, and assaulted his father-in-law as well. (The father-in-law survived.) He then drove to the police station and told police that he thought he had "killed some people."

Parks claimed he could not remember anything about the murder and attempted murder. Because he had a history of sleepwalking, his defense—and psychiatrist experts—claimed that he was asleep when he committed the acts. (It is unclear whether or not he was asleep while driving to the police station.) Parks was acquitted on both counts.

There have been many other homicide cases in which the defendant claimed that he or she was sleepwalking when harming the victim and therefore was innocent of the crime.

Sleepwalking, also called somnambulism, is a disorder that causes a person to walk or move around while asleep, with no conscious awareness or memory of doing so. It tends to run in families. It is very difficult to arouse a sleepwalker. The onset of somnambulism is usually before puberty. It is more common in boys than girls, and more common in children than in teens or adults.

Sleepwalkers navigate surprisingly well, considering that they are, well, not awake. Still, if you have a sleepwalker in the house, make sure to remove any objects that could be dangerous to the person, such as knives, firearms, blowtorches, etc. Keep doors and windows closed and locked so the person doesn't fall out or wander out. Ideally the person's bedroom should be on the ground floor.

In its most severe form, somnambulism can occur almost every night and involve physical injury to the sleepwalker, especially if he or she manages to exit the house. Sleepwalkers have even been known to walk through plate-glass windows. In such severe cases, medical treatment should be sought immediately.

SLEEP–RELATED EATING DISORDER

In a case reported in a *Sleep Review* magazine article by Allen Boone, a woman went to see a sleep specialist on the recommendation of her doctor. She had been feeling noticeably drowsy during the day. She had a hard time concentrating at work. She had gained a lot of weight, despite careful eating habits.

The woman reported one interesting thing: In the mornings she would often wake up to a sink full of dirty dishes and cookie crumbs. But she had no idea how they had gotten there.

It turned out that she suffered from sleep-related eating disorder, which is related to sleepwalking. People with this disorder get up in the middle of the night and eat, even going so far as to prepare elaborate meals. They have no memory of doing this the next morning.

This disorder is different from nocturnal eating syndrome. With this syndrome, people get up in the middle of the night because they have an overwhelming urge to snack. But they are fully awake and conscious the entire time.

Patients with sleep-related eating disorder are often totally indiscriminate about what they munch on in the wee hours. They have been known to eat cat food, salt and sugar "sand-wiches," raw bacon, and "smoothies" made of coffee grounds and milk. They have also been known to eat cigarette butts, plastic lids from margarine containers, and ammonia cleaning solution. One person even claimed to butter aluminum cans and try to eat them in her sleep.

People with this syndrome are also indiscriminate about *how* they eat. They can turn the kitchen upside down, eat uncooked spaghetti with their hands, and so forth. One woman reportedly chowed down on pancakes in the middle of the night while naked.

Often, the only way they know that something is wrong is because of an eyewitness or because they will wake up to find "evidence" of their middle-of-the-night food orgies. One woman reported that she often found peanut butter and spaghetti stains all over her pajamas in the mornings. Others have reported more serious aftereffects, such as lacerations, cuts, and burns from cooking while asleep.

SLEEP TALKING

"Quit using the goddamn bowl for banging like that—quit it now! Get the hell out of here! Go on! That's about four times this morning that I have told you. I don't know if you're that deaf or that dumb, which . . . goddamn continuously . . . what the hell are you looking for, a wall-eye?"

These strange words were spoken by a man while he was completely asleep. They were recorded for a video on sleep disorders and reported by Chip Brown in a February 3, 2003, *New York Times* article on the subject.

The man in question suffers from a parasomnia known as sleep talking, characterized by speaking in one's sleep, whether it's a few mumbled words or the entire text of the Declaration of Independence. The sleeper does not remember this behavior in the morning. The condition tends to be temporary, and may be related to stress, illness, or other, more serious sleep disorders.

Sleep talking is relatively harmless, unless of course the sleeper is disclosing state secrets or spilling the details of an illicit affair. Indeed, on one sleep-related Web site, a man wrote to the site's advice columnist saying that he was constantly talking about other women in his sleep and getting in trouble with his girlfriend, whom he claimed to love. The columnist wrote back and recommended sleep aids and strategies to achieve deeper sleep (which would "paralyze" his sleep-talking habits)—or, in lieu of that, act on what seemed to be his subconscious wish to be a free man and date other women.

SLEEP TERRORS

Have you ever woken up in the middle of the night screaming in terror, perhaps even struggling to escape an invisible
attacker? You may have been suffering from sleep terrors. Sleep
terrors are characterized by sudden awakening followed by
an overwhelming feeling of fear that can cause the person to
react physically, even violently. Those suffering from sleep terrors have been known to hurt themselves or other people. As
with other parasomnias, victims of sleep terrors have no memory of the episode the next day. Sleep terror is also known as
incubus, severe autonomic discharge, night terror, and pavor
nocturnus.

REM MOVEMENT DISORDER

During a normal REM cycle, the sleeper is temporarily "paralyzed" and unable to move or be moved. About the only things
moving are the eyes (ergo the term *rapid eye movement*) and the
busy dream activities inside the sleeper's brain.

However, when a person is suffering from REM movement
disorder, the paralysis is partially or wholly absent, allowing
the sleeper to "act out" dreams physically. This can lead to
violent behavior and injuries to the sleeper or others, and is
very bad news if the sleeper happens to be dreaming about the
battle scenes in *The Lord of the Rings.* Indeed, the sleep-talker in
Chip Brown's article once had a dream that he was trying to
snap a deer's neck. He woke suddenly to the sound of his wife

yelling. He realized that he was in bed with her and that it was *her* neck he was in the process of snapping, not a deer's. Fortunately, his wife survived the incident.

SEXUAL BEHAVIORS DURING SLEEP

A woman noticed that her husband had turned into a nocturnal animal. He had recently developed the habit of initiating unusually aggressive sex with her while in a state of slumber— groping, biting, and so forth. For a while she thought that he was just *pretending* to be asleep. But eventually she realized that he really *was* asleep because the next day he never seemed to remember what had happened the previous night.

Sexual behaviors during sleep (SBS) is a possible new addition to the parasomnia family, although it has not been officially characterized as such. SBS is the initiation of sexual activity— sometimes forceful, aggressive, or otherwise uncharacteristic of the person—while asleep.

Sometimes, partners of SBS sufferers grow to enjoy the nighttime encounters. In other cases, however, rape or brutality can be involved, as well as other inappropriate behaviors such as incest or sex with children.

SBS sufferers often don't report their symptoms to their physicians out of guilt and embarrassment. Women as well as men can suffer from SBS. The sexual activity during sleep can be with a partner or entirely solo; reported cases of masturbatory activity during SBS episodes are often violent and compulsive in nature. Some SBS cases are fairly mild, however, and simply involve loud sexual moaning during sleep.

MULTIPLE SLEEP DISORDERS

Some people suffer from multiple sleep disorders, which lends credence to the idea that certain sleep disorders may have common underlying causes and other connective factors. For example, a twenty-seven-year-old man had a history of sleep-walking from the time he was nine years old. As an adult, he also suffered from dream enactment—REM movement disorder—which led to physical injuries to himself, his wife, and their baby. These episodes happened about once a week.

Then, from his early twenties on, the man began initiating sex with his wife while he was asleep. He would manage to achieve complete sexual intercourse and not remember a thing the next day. Sleep researchers asked the man if he would consent to being videotaped during the night. He refused.

NARCOLEPSY

Narcolepsy is not a parasomnia but is rather a non–sleep-time sleep disorder. Narcoleptics suffer from the need to sleep a lot and at inopportune times. Narcoleptic sleep attacks can strike anytime: while driving, while carrying on a conversation, while walking down the street. They can last a few seconds or over half an hour.

Narcolepsy affects the person by messing with the part of the brain that regulates sleep and wakefulness. The result is the sudden, inappropriate onset of REM sleep, even while going sixty-five down the Mass. Pike.

Other characteristics of narcolepsy include cataplexy, which involves a sudden loss of muscle control, which can make narcoleptics fall to the ground or drop a package. Narcoleptics can also suffer from sleep paralysis, which makes them unable to move or speak as they transition from sleep to wakefulness or from wakefulness to sleep. Another symptom that can manifest itself during these transitions is "hypnagogic hallucinations," which are vivid, dreamlike images that can sometimes be nightmarish and terrifying.

No cure currently exists for narcolepsy, although stimulants and antidepressants can help manage the symptoms.

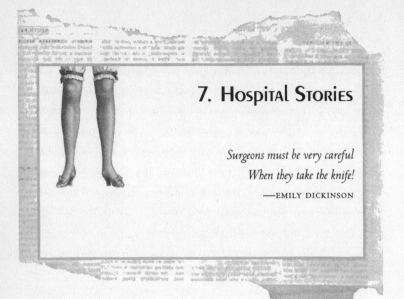

7. Hospital Stories

Surgeons must be very careful
When they take the knife!

—EMILY DICKINSON

THOSE OF US WHO ARE ADDICTED TO *ER* AND OTHER medical shows know that in hospitals, everything that can happen, seems to happen. Hospitals can be real-life theaters for life's richest comedies and darkest tragedies.

This chapter will cover both ends of the spectrum. On the humorous side, there are anecdotes of patients with unusual, laugh-out-loud problems and doctors with unusual, laugh-out-loud responses.

On the grimmer side, there are anecdotes of hospital procedures gone terribly wrong.

In the best of all possible worlds, operations and other medical procedures would always be A Sure Thing. Doctors would always remove the right limbs, take out the right organs, and in general never, ever make a mistake or leave surgical tools in the body cavity.

The same applies to medical procedures outside the OR. When it comes to a patient's health and welfare—to that fine line between life and death—doctors, nurses, and other medical personnel cannot afford to make even the slightest wrong move.

And yet, they do. According to a 1999 report by the National Academy of Sciences' Institute of Medicine, anywhere from 44,000 to 98,000 patients die as a result of mistakes made in hospitals each year. Cases of patients receiving the wrong medications, the wrong doses of chemotherapy, and worse are alarmingly common.

One medical-mistake category, "wrong-site surgeries," such as operating on the wrong side of the brain, has been a nationally recognized problem since the mid-1990s. Many of these errors tend to take place in freestanding (not attached to a hospital) surgical clinics, which often have smaller staffs than hospitals. In order to avoid these tragic errors, the Joint Commission on Accreditation of Healthcare Organizations (JCAHO), which accredits a majority of U.S. hospitals, created a set of "national patient safety goals." Among the goals is a recommendation to patients that they ask their surgeon to mark the surgical site before the operation—just to be sure both doctor and patient are on the same page.

Of course, mistakes aren't the only causes of medical mishaps. Accidents happen. The dice can roll the wrong way. A patient can find himself among the unfortunate .01 percent in a procedure that has a fatality risk of .01 percent.

This chapter includes several striking examples of medicine-gone-wrong, whether by accident, negligence, or unfortunate circumstances—or by a patient's self-inflicted injury, as you will see in the final anecdote.

THE CASE OF THE KILLER RAT

In Tegucigalpa, Honduras, over a dozen hospital patients at the Mario Catarino Rivasto Hospital died because of a little rat.

According to the Weird But True! Web site, the rat in question had a feeding frenzy on the hospital's electrical system one night and chewed through a number of wires. There was a short circuit in the ICU as a result. The patients didn't receive the oxygen they needed and died. Their bodies were discovered by nurses the next morning.

THE CASE OF THE POOR PATIENT

"Bizarre Tales from A&E" (short for Accident and Emergency Medicine) on the BBC News Online Web site contains a strange tale of mistaken identity. A man was admitted to the OR but died before he could be treated. One of the nurses took off his jacket and went through the pockets to ascertain his identity. She finally found something and announced, "His name is John Stevens."

Hearing this, the anesthesiologist said, "*I'm* John Stevens. And that's my jacket!"

THE CASE OF THE WRONG REMEDY

In another BBC News Online story, an elderly man appeared at the OR with a painful problem. He had been bothered by his inability to pee in a straight line. So he had decided to improve his aim by inserting a portion of a ballpoint pen into his member to "straighten things out." He needed medical assistance to get the pen out again.

THE CASE OF THE WOULD-BE SANTA CLAUS

The BBC News Online Web site also has a tale about a man who decided to play Santa Claus one holiday. He climbed onto his roof and decided to go down the chimney with the Christmas presents. In order to secure himself, he tied a rope around his waist; the other end was tied to the bumper of his car.

Unfortunately, his unknowing wife got into the car and drove off. Fortunately, the man survived with minor injuries.

THE CASE OF THE WRONG KIDNEY

Two Welsh surgeons were put on trial for the death of seventy-year-old Graham Reeves, who died five weeks after the surgeons removed the wrong kidney. In January of 2000, Mr. Reeves had gone into Prince Philip Hospital in Llanelli in order to have his diseased right kidney removed, and signed a consent form to that effect. But owing to what was described as a "fateful chain of events," the head surgeon, John Roberts, and his team removed the healthy left kidney instead. Later on the day of the operation, Mr. Reeves underwent a second operation in an effort to try to salvage his diseased remaining kidney. He was transferred to another hospital later on for dialysis but developed septicemia, a blood infection, and eventually died.

Both surgeons were cleared of the charges.

THE CASE OF THE WRONG PATIENT

In his June 8, 2002, *New York Times* article "Oops, Wrong Patient: Journal Takes on Medical Mistakes," Dennis Grady described a new series of articles about medical errors. The series was being published in the journal *Annals of Internal Medicine.*

One of the articles focused on two patients with similar names who were in the hospital, referred to pseudonymously as Mrs. Morris and Mrs. Morrison. Mrs. Morris was there for an operation for an aneurysm in her skull, and Mrs. Morrison for an invasive procedure to check out her heart.

Due to a series of mix-ups, partially having to do with the similarity of the names, Mrs. Morris was taken to the OR, opened up at the groin, had a tube inserted in an artery and snaked up into her heart, and more—before the doctor realized that he was working on the wrong patient. Not only had he subjected her to an invasive procedure but he had exposed her to numerous unnecessary risks: infection, bleeding, stroke, and heart attack. He was supposed to have been working on Mrs. Morrison all along.

The wronged Mrs. Morris was more than gracious about the whole episode. Not only did she not sue, she also acknowledged that at least she knew her heart was healthy.

THE CASE OF THE WRONG LEG

In 1995, a fifty-one-year-old man named Willie King went into the University Community Hospital in Tampa, Florida, to get his diseased right leg amputated. According to various news reports, the surgeon got "right" and "left" mixed up and removed the wrong leg.

Mr. King, a diabetic, suffered from progressive vascular disease in both legs. His left leg, in fact, was not much better than his right. But he had asked that his right leg be removed because it was causing him more pain and discomfort.

After the incident, Mr. King sued the hospital. The case was settled privately.

THE CASE OF THE STRANGE BIRTHDAY

A Veterans Administration hospital in Kansas City, Missouri, issued two "birth announcements" in 1998. The births in question had nothing to do with babies—not *human* babies, anyway. Instead, it was discovered that maggots had hatched in the noses of two comatose patients.

"We learned from that incident and took action to make sure it doesn't happen again," Pat Landon, the hospital's director of facilities, was quoted as saying in an Associated Press article.

The article goes on to explain that according to a report issued by the journal *Archives in Internal Medicine*, the hospital was infested with mice and flies. Hospital employees in the director's suite claimed that mice would sometimes dash over their feet. The mouse infestation apparently began when the hospital cafeteria and food storage areas were erroneously dropped from a cleaning list. The mice moved in, then happily migrated to other parts of the hospital.

A pest-control contractor was hired to exterminate the mice in July of 1998 but did not remember to clean up all the dead mice. This oversight reportedly led to the subsequent fly infestation, since flies like to lay their eggs on dead mice.

The aforementioned baby maggots were found in the nostrils of one comatose patient on July 22, 1998. The second comatose patient became a proud parent sometime on or before September 30, 1998.

THE CASE OF THE FORGOTTEN SPONGES

Maria Tovias sued a hospital in Texas for complications following her abdominal surgery in 1999. Tovias claimed that she had "continuing abdominal pain" and "fluid buildup" nine months after the surgery.

According to a *National Law Journal* item posted on the Jester's Courtroom Archive Web site, it turned out that Tovias's nasty symptoms were caused by a sponge that had been left in her stomach when the laparotomy incision was sewn up. The hospital and surgeon claimed innocence, saying that all their surgical sponges were accounted for. They said they could not explain how this mysterious "extra" sponge had ended up in her stomach. The jury found in Tovias's favor and awarded her nearly half a million dollars.

According to a January 2003 study published in *The New England Journal of Medicine*, Tovias's case represents a much larger and very serious problem. The study claims that on average, surgery tools such as sponges and clamps are left in 1,500 American patients per year.

THE CASE OF THE BIZARRE HAIRDO

According to an AP article, surgeons were amazed to see twenty-five-year-old William Bartron of Lehighton, Pennsylvania, arrive at the hospital with at least a dozen inch-long nails sticking out of his scalp. It turned out that Bartron had cut off his hand with a power saw (by accident). In order to distract himself from the excruciating pain while awaiting help, he had shot himself in the head repeatedly with a nail gun.

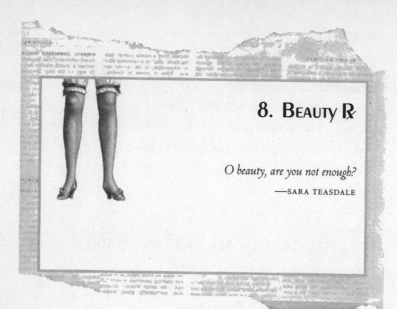

8. Beauty Rx

O beauty, are you not enough?

—SARA TEASDALE

WE LIVE IN A "BEFORE AND AFTER" SOCIETY THAT IS OB-
sessed with beauty, youth, and sexual attractiveness. For those
of us who aren't naturally blessed with those attributes, or
want more (or less) of what we have, there are all sorts of
medical interventions that can tweak us in the right direction.
Whether we're talking bigger breasts, flatter abs, a more mas-
culine jaw, or fewer wrinkles, there's something for everyone.

Of course, these procedures come at a cost. Not only can
they be expensive and time-consuming, but once a person is on
the hamster wheel of cosmetic enhancement, she (and increasingly, he) just might be stuck there—for life. Worse yet, such
procedures can saddle a person with various unwanted side
effects and aftereffects, the worst of which can be illness, permanent disfigurement, or death.

On the other hand, proponents claim that there's nothing wrong with looking better or feeling more sexually vibrant, which can have positive ripple effects on romance, professional success, financial success, and overall sense of well-being.

Not surprisingly, the phenomenon of cosmetic enhancement didn't start with breast implants and Botox.

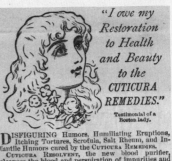

"I owe my Restoration to Health and Beauty to the CUTICURA REMEDIES."

Testimonial of a Boston lady.

DISFIGURING Humors, Humiliating Eruptions, Itching Tortures, Scrofula, Salt Rheum, and Infantile Humors cured by the CUTICURA REMEDIES.
CUTICURA RESOLVENT, the new blood purifier, cleanses the blood and perspiration of impurities and poisonous elements, and thus removes the *cause.*
CUTICURA, the great Skin Cure, instantly allays Itching and Inflammation, clears the Skin and Scalp, heals Ulcers and Sores, and restores the Hair.
CUTICURA SOAP, an exquisite Skin Beautifier and Toilet Requisite, prepared from CUTICURA, is indispensable in treating Skin Diseases, Baby Humors, Skin Blemishes, Chapped and Oily Skin.
CUTICURA REMEDIES are absolutely pure, and the only infallible Blood Purifiers and Skin Beautifiers.
Sold everywhere. Price, Cuticura, 50 cents; Soap, 25 cents; Resolvent, $1.
POTTER DRUG AND CHEMICAL CO., BOSTON, MASS.

Women have been doing this stuff—or have been *forced* to do this stuff by the dictates of culture and society—for thousands of years. "The Price of Perfection," an article by Robin Marantz Henig, contains some interesting historical examples. During the Renaissance, fashionable European women gave themselves high foreheads, considered beautiful at the time, by plucking their hairs one by one and extending their natural hairlines back to the crowns of their heads. An alternative to plucking was the use of poultices that were made from a mixture of vinegar and cat feces, or from a substance known as quicklime, which could rip up the skin as well. The Mangbettu people in Africa wrapped the heads of their baby girls in giraffe hide; this was done to make their heads long and cone-shaped, which was considered to be extremely attractive. Until World War Two, Chinese infant girls of the upper classes had their feet bound. Though very painful and crippling, this practice gave them tiny feet—often just three or so inches long—that were considered very feminine by upper-class Chinese men.

In this chapter you will learn more about what happens when beauty meets medicine—cases in which medicine has been employed for the purpose of beautification and, conversely, in which beautification has led to dire or disastrous medical results.

ARSENIC AND OLD LACE

Since the dawn of history, women have been seeking ways to achieve radiant, beautiful skin. Unfortunately, simple cleansers and creams never seemed to do the trick. Indeed, some women have always sought extreme, dangerous, and even deadly treatments in their pursuit of the perfect complexion.

According to "The Price of Perfection," in Elizabethan England, women tried to whiten their skin with ceruse, which was a combination of vinegar and lead. Queen Elizabeth I used so much of the corrosive solution that it eventually ate permanent pits into her skin, leading her to ban all mirrors from her castles.

By the mid-1800s, women discovered other dangerous methods of skin-whitening such as swallowing vinegar or painting their faces with enamel.

An extremely popular beauty tonic at that time was arsenic. Victorian women actually ingested small amounts of arsenic in order to achieve their lovely, deathly pale complexions. Not all of them were meticulous at measuring, however; some reportedly died from a slow accumulation of the substance in their systems.

As it turns out, arsenic is one of the nastier poisons in the poison universe. It can be swallowed as a powder or inhaled as a dust or gas.

The *Encyclopedia Britannica* lists the symptoms of arsenic poisoning as nausea, vomiting, severe gastric distress, and burning sensations in the throat and mouth. In cases of chronic arsenic poisoning, the symptoms may include hair loss, diarrhea, constipation, streaking of the fingernails, and skin changes such as scaling or discoloration.

Because arsenic does not break down, it can be found in the victim's urine, fingernails, and hair.

Originally identified as an element in the seventeenth century, arsenic came to be used in a compound called Paris green, which was developed in the 1770s by a Swedish apothecary and chemist, Carl Scheele. Paris green (also called Scheele's green), copper arsenite, was used as a pigment to color fabrics, wallpaper, and paints. According to Victoria King's article "Arsenic," people reportedly became sick from living in houses papered with wallpaper containing Paris green, but its hazardous effects were not recognized until the late nineteenth century.

When Napoleon died in 1821, the official cause of his death was listed as stomach cancer. An autopsy revealed that his hair contained trace amounts of arsenic. He could have ingested the arsenic by eating seafood, since seawater contains arsenic. Another theory is that the arsenic came from his home, which was decorated with Paris green wallpaper.

King explains that in addition to being a beauty aid, arsenic was a common way to kill off rich relatives and boring husbands during the nineteenth century. Some people even referred to arsenic as "inheritance powder." For one thing, it was readily available and easy to administer. For example, flypaper contained arsenic. When it was soaked in water, the resulting toxic tincture could be surreptitiously mixed with foods and beverages.

In the eighteenth century there was a Frenchman who used arsenic in an ingenious way to kill his rich, beautiful wife . . . then the next wife . . . then the next wife . . . and on and on. During sex, he wore a thin goatskin condom upon which he had applied a hefty dose of arsenic. During the act, the arsenic would be absorbed in the women's vaginas and kill them shortly afterward. The Frenchman was eventually caught by the authorities, who became suspicious that he managed to "lose" so many wives. He was eventually hanged.

It is possible to develop a tolerance for arsenic (although this suggests the question: Why go there?). There were so-called arsenic eaters throughout history who ingested arsenic daily, presumably to prove some sort of point. Members of the Hell Fire Club of Regency and Victorian England frequently made a practice of playing "chicken" with arsenic and other poisons.

These days, arsenic is continuing to do its damage. It has been linked to cancer of the bladder, lung, skin, kidney, liver, prostate gland, and nasal passages. Heated debates rage within the scientific, medical, and environmental policy communities about acceptable levels of arsenic in our drinking water.

BELLADONNA

Yes, it's a Stevie Nicks song. It is also a plant, one that enhanced the beauty of women—the ones who survived it, that is.

The word *belladonna* means "beautiful woman" in Italian. During the Renaissance, women would apply belladonna extract to their eyes in order to dilate their pupils and keep them dilated, giving their eyes more depth and brilliance, which was a desirable trait.

Belladonna also goes by the names *deadly nightshade, banewort, naked lady lily,* and a number of other monikers. Modern experts believe that the long-term effects of belladonna eyedrops may have been a predisposition to glaucoma and possibly blindness. If belladonna is taken internally, it can paralyze the parasympathetic nervous system and bring on hallucinations, fever, and death faster than you can say "Stop draggin' my heart around."

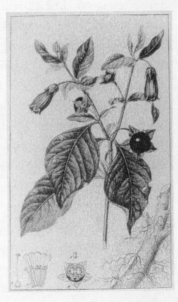

Remember *Psycho*? According to the Movie Mistakes Web site: "When Janet Leigh is shown lying dead on the floor, there is a close-up of her open eye. The pupil is contracted to a pinpoint (obviously due to the bright lighting) where it should have been dilated. After the film was released, Hitchcock heard from several ophthalmologists who pointed this out and suggested he use belladonna eyedrops in the eyes of 'dead' people in the future, as the chemical prevents the pupils from contracting."

MODERN–DAY SKIN TREATMENTS

Of course, we're so much smarter now. Take the botulinum toxin (which causes botulism), for example.

The botulinum toxin is one of the nastiest, most danger-ous poisons in the world. Botulism, which is usually contracted from eating contaminated food, can cause major damage to the nervous system and subsequent paralysis. If the respiratory muscles are paralyzed, death by suffocation can be the result. As if that weren't bad enough, the botulinum toxin has been mentioned on the news as a potential bioterrorism agent.

All that being said . . . Botox injections are a popular new skin treatment, and Botox is the best-known brand name for a type of botulinum toxin. Proponents claim that Botox injec-tions, administered by a cosmetologist or other professional, can eliminate unsightly wrinkles by paralyzing selected facial muscles. Botox is only effective on wrinkles that are muscular in origin, such as those between the brows and crow's-feet, the ones you get from repetitive facial expressions. It is not effective on other types of wrinkles, such as those caused by sun damage.

According to the *University of California, Berkeley Wellness Letter,* the amount of botulinum toxin in a Botox injection is too small actually to cause the disease. Still, people have reported side effects such as redness, bruising, pain, mild swelling, double vision, a drooping eyelid or brow, and temporary paralysis of surrounding muscles, which can sometimes result in a clownlike "frozen smile" look.

You may have heard of Botox parties, in which a bunch of women get together at someone's house, sip sangrias, crank up the Mariah Carey tunes, and take turns receiving Botox injections from a doctor (or someone who plays a doctor) who has kindly consented to make a house call. Needless to say, it's probably best and safest to get the treatments at the office of a licensed dermatologist or other physician.

Incidentally, Botox has other uses besides making those nasty wrinkles disappear. It is sometimes injected into the armpits of people who have excessive sweating problems. Botox also appears successful in helping people who suffer from incontinence: The injections prevent overactive bladder muscles from spasming. Studies are under way to look at Botox as a treatment for hemorrhoids and migraine.

There are many other popular modern-day skin treatments besides Botox. Chemical peels involve the application of some type of acidic chemical to the skin that is later "peeled" off. The strongest peel, which might contain the chemical phenol, goes after serious wrinkles, severe sun damage, and other deep-down problems. Regional nerve blocks are given to anesthetize the "work area," and the patient's heart must be monitored during the entire procedure, since the chemical can damage the heart (as well as the liver and kidneys). Possible side effects of chemical-peel procedures include redness, irritation, scarring, swelling, allergic reaction, infection, and variations in pigmentation.

Laser resurfacing is a more *Star Wars* approach to obtaining baby-butt-smooth skin. This technique, which should not be employed at home, targets a number of skin problems: stretch marks, birthmarks, age spots, fine wrinkles, spider veins, and more. Different types of lasers go after different problems. Possible side effects and aftereffects include redness for up to six months, tenderness, skin peeling, pigmentation changes, scarring, infection, and crusting.

Another modern route to beautiful skin is "permanent makeup." For those women who are tired of having to apply that Maybelline every single darned morning, they can have their makeup tattooed on permanently. The most popular choices are lip tattoos, eyebrow tattoos, and eyeliner tattoos.

The tattooing is best done in the office of a cosmetologist or plastic surgeon, not by Bud, the chain-smoking, Harley-riding tattoo guy around the corner. In addition to temporary swelling and scabbing, there are several, more serious risks associated with this procedure. A person can have an allergic reaction to the dyes (which, incidentally, are not regulated by the FDA). There is the possibility of contracting hepatitis and other infections.

THE PERFECT BODY

Before Jenny Craig, Weight Watchers, power yoga, and Pilates, there were all sorts of interesting techniques for weight loss.

According to "The Price of Perfection," in seventeenth-century England, overweight women were advised to try blood-letting (bleeding with leeches) in order to get rid of excess fat.

In the 1930s, women swallowed tapeworms to achieve the same effect.

Women today have a range of options for achieving just the right figure; unfortunately, some of them seem just as barbaric as using leeches and tapeworms. Take liposuction, for example. With this procedure, a woman literally gets her fat sucked out of her with a high-tech vacuum cleaner.

Liposuction is a procedure that permanently removes fat deposits from various areas of the body, including the thighs, abdomen, and buttocks, and, less commonly, the face, neck, chest, ankles, and breasts. A wee little incision is made into the skin, and then a thin, hollow metal rod is wedged into the incision. The surgeon swishes the metal rod back and forth as suction is applied.

After the procedure, the patient sometimes dons a girdle-like garment in order to reduce swelling. Recovery can take several weeks, and final results may not be evident for several months or even a year. The list of possible risks is rather long, and includes swelling, irritation, bruising, bleeding, infection, dimpling, dents, uneven contour, pigmentation changes, and blood clots.

As with other types of cosmetic surgeries, men are seeking liposuction treatments almost as frequently as women. Realizing that looking younger and buffer isn't just for the ladies anymore, men are spending record dollars being surgically sculpted, smoothed, and more. The three most popular areas for the guys to look to liposuction to fix are the love handles, abdomen, and neck. Some surgeons use liposuction to help men with gynecomastia, a disorder that afflicts males with large breasts.

Another modern shortcut to weight loss is a procedure called abdominoplasty. Commonly known as a "tummy tuck," this procedure involves multiple steps: liposuctioning of abdominal fat, then tightening and repairing abdominal muscles, then removing excessive skin from the abdomen.

There are three types of abdominoplasty: the mini, the modified, and the full (kind of like coffee-cup sizes at Starbucks). The mini is for those whose fat is concentrated below the navel area; you get a small incision in the pubic hairline. With the modified, you get a bigger incision, below the navel. With the full, which is for people with fat above and below the navel, you get a big, happy smiley-face incision from hip to hip.

Women who have saggy bellies due to pregnancy are fond of the abdominoplasty procedure. However, women who are contemplating a future pregnancy or pregnancies are usually advised to wait to have this procedure, since tummy-tucked abdominal muscles can separate when put under strain by pregnancy.

There is much talk and rumor about a procedure in which women have several ribs removed in order to achieve an hourglass figure. Hopefully this is just talk and rumor, since most reputable doctors denounce this practice as dangerous and horrific.

Still, women obviously do go to extremes to get rid of pounds and inches. Some of them, unfortunately, suffer dire consequences.

In 2002, a Detroit city councilwoman, Brenda Scott, died after undergoing weight-reduction surgery at the Port Huron Hospital. She had undergone a new procedure called lap-band adjustable gastric banding, in which a noose is tightened around the stomach in order to limit food consumption. Scott, who weighed more than three hundred pounds, died three days after the procedure from an infection caused by a stomach perforation. Her death was ruled an accident by the medical examiner.

The FDA approved this procedure in June of 2001. At that time, it had been performed on more than 90,000 people in other countries, mostly Europe.

BREASTS, BREASTS, BREASTS

Throughout the years and around the world, there have been different standards as to what constitutes "attractive" female breasts. According to "The Price of Perfection," in ancient Greece, a woman's breasts were tightly bound and hidden from sight. Among the Circassian women of Eurasia, young girls were tightly wrapped in leather clothes from the beginning of adolescence until the time they were married to keep their breasts from growing. On her wedding night, a girl's leather garment was slashed with a hunting knife by her husband. In America in the 1920s, flat chests were very much in vogue, driving some women to literally squash their breasts against their rib cages and bind them there with elastic.

At the other end of the spectrum, many societies appreciate the charms of large—*very* large—breasts. For those women who were blessed with less than ample bosoms, breast enhancement became the thing to do.

In 1903, a Chicago surgeon named Charles Miller opened a cosmetic-surgery practice. He experimented with various

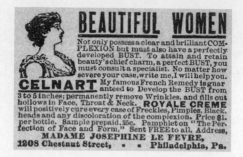

surgical breast-enlargement techniques, and was known to
open up women's breasts and insert such wacky substances as
celluloid particles, braided silk, silk floss, and vegetable ivory.

Over the next few decades, breast augmentation surgery
became more refined. One of the first customers for modern-
day breast augmentation was Carol Doda, a former plum picker
and file clerk who became a topless San Francisco cocktail
waitress. According to the Web site article "Carol Doda and
the Topless Era" by Marsha Garland, in 1964, Doda underwent twenty weeks of liquid-silicone treatments, which at the
time cost $2,000. Now a whopping 44DD, she had them
insured for $1.5 million by Lloyds of London. In 1974, Har-
vard University named Doda "Business Person of the Year." In
the 1980s, after her topless days were over, she went on to
launch a lingerie company as well as a fantasy phone line, Tele-
Doda.

In 1992 the FDA restricted the use of silicone implants in
breast augmentation procedures. This restriction occurred because many women were experiencing serious health problems
as a result of rupturing and leaking implants.

The other type of implants, used today, is made of saline,

or saltwater. Risks associated with saline implants include ruptured or deflated implants, infection, scarring, nerve damage, and hardening of the tissues surrounding the implant—as well as romantic partners complaining about hard "titanium titties" (referring to the metallic element) and disgruntled strangers muttering, "Are those real?"

Another problem with breast augmentation procedures is their cost, which can be fairly high. Of course, there are stories of women who've gotten their procedures paid for by appreciative men. According to a *Florida Times-Union* item posted on the Jester's Courtroom Web site, a waitress at the Hooters in Jacksonville Landing, Florida, wanted to enlarge her breasts but couldn't afford the cost. Fortunately for her, one of her regular customers—Somchart "Nick" Fungcharoen, a retired engineer from the Army Corps of Engineers—offered to pay for the operation. "She served me and was nice to me" was the reason Fungcharoen gave.

Later, Fungcharoen sued the former waitress—now an officer with the Jacksonville sheriff's office—for $3,940 in small claims court. He claimed that this amount, which he charged to his credit card in order to pay for her procedure, was only a loan.

She countered by saying that there was never any mention of a loan, and that during the months after her operation, while she still worked at Hooters (and while he still visited her there, as a customer) he never mentioned wanting repayment.

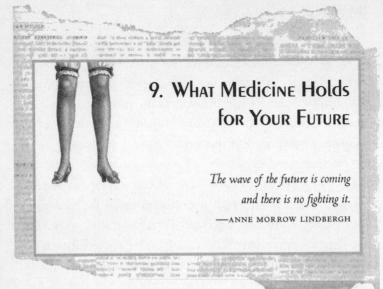

9. What Medicine Holds for Your Future

The wave of the future is coming and there is no fighting it.

—ANNE MORROW LINDBERGH

"*We can rebuild him. We have the technology.*"

Those memorable lines from *The Six Million Dollar Man*, that thrillingly hokey 1970s show that I was glued to every Friday night, used to be the stuff of scriptwriters and science-fiction geeks.

But no longer. These days, new advances in medicine and biotechnology far surpass anything those wild, wacky kids in the entertainment industry could ever have dreamed up.

Indeed, thanks to modern medicine, incurable diseases are becoming curable . . . women are giving birth in their fifties and sixties . . . and scientists are predicting life expectancies to double. Previously out-there concepts like bioengineered human tissue, cryogenics, and human cloning are becoming reality.

In this final chapter, you will read about some of the latest and greatest breakthroughs in medicine—as well as what may be just over the horizon.

ARTIFICIAL EMOTIONAL CREATURE PROJECT

One potential strategy for enhancing the emotional and physical health of our nation's elderly and other needy populations is pet robots, or "artificial emotional creatures." Developed by Japanese scientists as part of an ongoing artificial intelligence project, these barking 'bots were designed to interact with humans, engage their affections, learn new behaviors, and more.

One version of the artificial emotional creature is Paro, a robotic seal. Paro was created by Dr. Takanori Shibata, a research scientist who specializes in bio-robotics and artificial intelligence. He is affiliated with the Massachusetts Institute of Technology as well as various research institutions in Japan, including the Human Friendly System Research Group at the Intelligent Systems Institute in Tsukuba.

Paro was specifically designed to be a therapeutic robot. According to an artificial intelligence Web site called Generation 5: "It reacts when it is touched, generates heat, and even has antibacterial fur!"

STEM CELLS GALORE

According to many experts, stem cell research is *the* medical wave of the future, promising not only to regenerate damaged cells but also to *grow* replacement organs. We're talking a brand-new liver, kidney, heart—all from some itty-bitty cells that are hanging out in your body anyway. Scientists believe that some-day, stem cells will provide cures for heart disease, diabetes, and Parkinson's disease, among other things.

The science of stem-cell therapy falls under the category of "regenerative" or "reparative" medicine. Stem cells are differ-ent from other cells because they are capable of very long-term self-renewal (by replicating over and over again); because they are unspecialized; and because under certain conditions, they can be persuaded to become specialized, differentiated cells: They can morph into heart cells that help the heart beat, into pancreas cells that produce insulin, and so forth. They are, in essence, blank-slate cells that can be transformed into millions of heart cells or pancreas cells or whatever other kind of cell is needed.

There are two kinds of animal and human stem cells that scientists are working on: embryonic stem cells and adult stem cells. And therein lies the controversy. Some critics focus on serious bioethical issues raised by the use of cells from embryos for scientific purposes, whether the origin of the embryos is in vitro fertilization, an aborted pregnancy, or a clone (which has not yet been created successfully, even though many have tried). It remains to be seen how these issues will be sorted out; in the meantime, universities such as Stanford University in Palo Alto, California, are proceeding with major stem-cell research efforts, controversy or no.

TOOTH FARMING

Imagine a farmer planting seeds in a field and watching them grow into big, healthy, strapping teeth.

Tooth farming isn't *exactly* like that, but it's close. According to "The Ageless Body," an article by J. Alex Tarquinio, tooth farming is an experimental technology that involves using adult dental stem cells to grow and harvest biological teeth. Grown in petri dishes, these farmed teeth—if the technology proves to be successful—may replace dentures and implants someday.

Other experimental teeth technologies include decay-fighting "smart fillings" as well as a decay-fighting vaccine derived from—of all things—tobacco plants.

MAKE LIKE A SALAMANDER

And now, from a bunch of experts who think that they have a better idea than stem-cell technology . . .

Think about salamanders. Salamanders have the miraculous ability to naturally regenerate their legs, tails, and parts of their eyes and hearts all by themselves, with no help from stem-cell technologies or doctors of any kind.

Scientists believe that humans may be able to do this someday as well. According to a fascinating *New York Times* article by Andrew Pollack, some experts suggest that natural limb regeneration may be a better way to repair damaged organs than stem-cell technologies.

Scientists are still trying to learn the fine points of how salamanders and other creatures manage to regenerate parts of their bodies. Pollack uses the example of a red spotted newt to illustrate the broad strokes of the regeneration process: "When a limb is amputated in a newt, cells near the site of the injury lose their specialized properties and become 'de-differentiated' stem cells," he writes. "After forming a mound and multiplying, cells redifferentiate to form the numerous tissues needed to rebuild the limb. A month and a half later, the regeneration is complete." De-differentiation is a process by which "the animal, in effect, creates its own stem cells when they are needed," explains Pollack.

Although conceding that the "stem-cell school" is further along than they are, regeneration proponents believe that it's only a matter of time until they figure out how to make what works for the salamander work for us humans too. One advantage of natural limb regeneration over stem-cell therapy is that the former occurs naturally within the body, whereas the latter requires growing the cells in a laboratory and transplanting inside the body, running the risk of rejection.

Regeneration may be helped along in the future by drugs or genes, says Pollack. In fact, a new "natural regeneration" company has recently been formed, with millions of dollars of venture-capital support. The company, Hydra Biosciences, is dedicated to replicating natural generation in humans. Its name comes from the hydra, a creature that hangs out in ponds and manages to grow into two wholes when whacked in half. The hydra is in turn named after the Hydra, a mythical multi-headed beast that sprouted a few new heads every time some poor warrior chopped one off.

THE ART (ASSISTED REPRODUCTIVE TECHNOLOGIES) OF MAKING BABIES

Thanks to modern medicine, moms are getting older and older, leading to what could only be called the "diaper and denture generation."

In 2001, in Fréjus, France, sixty-two-year-old Jeanine Salomone became pregnant by means of in vitro fertilization and gave birth to a healthy baby. IVF entails combining sperm and egg in a laboratory so that the baby will be related genetically to one or both partners. The fertilized egg is then implanted in the woman's womb.

In this case, Salomone used a donated egg and her own brother's sperm, which meant that the woman's son was also her nephew. The doctors had no idea that the woman was using her brother's sperm. According to the British news Web site Ananova.com, the brother-sister team instigated this crafty plot in order to qualify for their mother's estate, which would have gone to their other siblings if the brother and sister had remained childless.

This financially minded new mom is not the oldest woman to give birth, however. According to an April 9, 2003, report from the India Express news bureau, sixty-five-year-old Satyabhama Mahapatra of Orissa, India, gave birth to a baby boy the day before. Mahapatra and her husband, a retired schoolteacher, had been childless until then. The baby, who was born by caesarean section, was the result of an embryo from Mahapatra's niece.

Since the world's first "test-tube baby," Louise Brown, was born, having been conceived by means of IVF, there have been many advances in ART, or assisted reproductive technologies. Other ART procedures, many of which sound like *Star Trek: The Next Generation* terms, include gamete intrafallopian transfer (GIFT), zygote intrafallopian transfer (ZIFT), and pronuclear stage tubal transfer (PROST). For men whose sperm may not be operating at 100 percent, there is an ART procedure called intracytoplasmic sperm injection, which involves injecting one egg with one sperm only (versus lots and lots of the little swimming guys) in order to create an embryo.

Many people associate ART procedures with twins and triplets. Statistically, about two-thirds of ART births are single births, and most of the rest are multiple births, including twins, triplets, and so forth.

GENDER SELECTION

Science and technology often develop more quickly than the social and governmental policies that would govern them. Gender selection is yet another example.

One of the trickier aspects of ART procedures is being able to "pick" the sex of the baby. Embryos can be tested— boy or girl?—before implantation and selected on that basis.

In October 2001, the American Society for Reproductive Medicine (ASRM) issued a position paper suggesting that the use of technologies that can test the gender of embryos should be restricted, as ethical concerns have been raised regarding the practice of picking embryos for no other reason than their gender. Experts and nonexperts alike are worried about the implications of creating embryos for reproductive purposes, only to pick some and discard others on the basis of sex.

How far should two parents be permitted to go to make sure they have a boy instead of a girl, or vice versa? It's all very *Brave New World*—except it's not fiction anymore.

GENE CHIPS

No, this is not a new type of snack. Gene chips are special chips that can be used to treat tumors, especially aggressive ones.

Currently being tested on cancer patients, these tiny glass chips contain the DNA patterns of many genes from the human genome. During the procedure, RNA molecules are taken from the tumor in question and dyed with fluorescent dye. The molecules are then applied to the DNA chip. When the RNA finds its DNA "match" among the many choices, it will emit a shiny fluorescent glow. This tells doctors which of the tumor's genes are most active.

"IF I ONLY HAD A (TITANIUM) HEART"

In *The Wizard of Oz*, the Tin Man accompanied Dorothy to Oz so he could ask the wizard for a heart. He would have appreciated a new technology on the horizon: an artificial heart made of titanium and plastic.

The titanium-and-plastic AbioCor heart is manufactured by Abiomed, Inc., of Danvers, Massachusetts. Unlike previous artificial heart products such as the Jarvik-7, it is self-contained, meaning it has no wires or tubes or other parts sticking out of the chest and connecting to a big compressor device. The AbioCor runs on relatively light batteries that can be hidden under clothing.

The first recipient of the AbioCor heart, Robert Tools of Franklin, Kentucky, died in 2001, 151 days after the transplant operation. He and other recipients are part of a clinical trial by Abiomed. As of early 2003, ten U.S. patients had participated in the clinical trial. The longest-living heart recipient to date, Tom Christerson, died in February 2003 after surviving seventeen months with the heart.

This technology is still undergoing studies and testing. If the technology is given the green light, the titanium-and-plastic hearts will be welcome replacements for often scarce donor hearts.

FAKE BLOOD

Fake blood has always been useful for movies, plays, Halloween costumes, and kids freaking out the parents. But now fake blood is being used as a substitute for the real thing.

Blood substitutes are the wave of the future, promising ready-to-go, bountiful supplies of surrogate blood for hospital patients, accident victims, wounded soldiers, and others. One of the blood substitute products currently awaiting FDA approval is Hemopure, manufactured by Biopure of Cambridge, Massachusetts.

Hemopure is a polymerized hemoglobin solution derived from super-purified, super-processed cow's blood. It can delay or reduce the need for red blood cell transfusions. According to the Biopure Web site: "Hemopure is an oxygen therapeutic, or drug, consisting of chemically stabilized bovine hemoglobin formulated in a balanced salt solution. This stabilized hemoglobin circulates directly in plasma (the fluid part of blood) when infused, increasing oxygen diffusion to the body's tissues. The product is compatible with all blood types, can be stored for three years without refrigeration or special handling, and is purified through patented and proprietary techniques that are validated to remove potential contaminants, including infectious agents such as bacteria, viruses and transmissible spongiform encephalopathy (TSE) agents."

A blood substitute product such as Hemopure has several potential advantages over real blood. For one thing, while real blood has a shelf life of mere weeks, Biopure claims that Hemopure can last for three years. Biopure also states that, by its nature, Hemopure is suitable for any blood type: No more need to scramble for rare O-negative blood or any other blood type that might be in short supply.

Such advantages hold great promise for certain countries where safe blood is in short supply and for *all* countries when this may be the case. Hemopure has already been approved for use in South Africa and is being used in some hospitals there. Hemopure is also being tested in clinical trials in the United States and Europe.

IN CLONING (OR RATHER: IN CLOSING)

Of course this chapter—this whole book—could go on and on. Even as I write this, the Raelians—a Quebec-based group founded by Claude Vorihlon, aka Rael, who was allegedly charged with various earthly missions by a group of extraterrestrial visitors he met on a volcano in France—are claiming that they have produced cloned babies. Whether or not the Raelians will ever accomplish this (they have yet to cough up evidence of a cloned baby), some experts believe that successful human cloning is just a matter of time.

This author awaits with bated breath to see what other astonishing technologies and medical marvels continue to unfold in the twenty-first century.

Bibliography

INTRODUCTION

Krock, Lexi. "Accidental Discoveries," *Nova Online*, www.pbs.org/wgbh/nova/cancer/discoveries.html.

"Pain," *Encyclopedia Britannica*, 2003, Encyclopedia Britannica Premium Service, April 28, 2003, www.britannica.com/eb/article?eu=59461.

CHAPTER ONE

The Alton Museum of History and Art Web site, www.altonweb.com/history/wadlow.

Biddle, Wayne. *A Field Guide to Germs*, Knopf, 2002.

Cartwright, Frederick F., with Michael D. Biddiss, *Disease and History: The Influence of Disease in Shaping the Great Events of History*, Thomas W. Crowell, 1972.

The Centers for Disease Control and Prevention Web site, www.cdc.gov.

Defoe, Daniel. *A Journal of the Plague Year*, Charles E. Tuttle, 1994.

DeSalle, Rob, ed., *Epidemic! The World of Infectious Diseases*, New Press, 1999.

Gibson, Arthur C., "Leprosy," www.botgard.ucla.edu.

Goldmann, David R., ed., *The American College of Physicians Complete Home Medical Guide*, DK Publishing, 1999.

Gould, George M., and Walter L. Pyle, *Anomalies and Curiosities of Medicine*, Sydenham Publishers, 1937.

Hamill, Sam, trans., *The Essential Bashō*, Shambhala Publications, Inc., 1999.

Kantor, Norman F., *In the Wake of the Plague*, Free Press, 2001.

Knox, Ellis L., "The Black Death," http://history.boisestate.edu/westciv/plague/.

The Manlyweb Web site, www.manlyweb.com/realmen/R/Andre Rousimoff.html.

The Merck Manual of Diagnosis and Therapy, seventeenth edition, on-line edition, www.merck.com/pubs/mmanual.

Murphy, Wendy, *Orphan Diseases: New Hope for Rare Medical Conditions*, Twenty-first Century Books, 2002.

Musashi, "Fugu: The Deadly Delicacy," www.destroy-all-monsters.com/fugu.shtml.

The National Institutes of Health Web site, www.nih.gov.

The National Organization for Rare Disorders Web site, www.rarediseases.org.

Oldstone, Michael A. B., *Viruses, Plagues, and History*, Oxford University Press, 1998.

"Plague," *Encyclopedia Britannica*, 2003, Encyclopedia Britannica Premium Service, April 28, 2003, www.britannica.com/eb/article?eu=61809.

The Pubmed Web site of the National Library of Medicine, www. pubmed.org.

"Rabies: Risks and Responsibilities," Illinois Raptor Center, www. illinoisraptorcenter.org/rabies.html.

Roemmele, Jacqueline A., and Donna Batdorff, *Surviving the "Flesh-Eating Bacteria,"* Avery, 2000.

Stevens, Serita Deborah, with Anne Klarner, *Deadly Doses: A Writer's Guide to Poisons,* Writer's Digest Books, 1990.

Turkington, Carol, *The Poisons and Antidotes Sourcebook,* second edition, Checkmark Books, 1999.

The WebMD Web site, www.webmd.com.

The WholehealthMD Web site, www.wholehealthmd.com.

CHAPTER TWO

Balch, Phyllis A., *Prescription for Herbal Healing,* Avery, 2002.

"Banting, Sir Frederick Grant," *Encyclopedia Britannica,* 2003, Encyclopedia Britannica Premium Service, May 23, 2003, www.britannica. com/eb/article?eu=13372.

Bean, Matt, "Doctor: Victim Injected with Insulin," February 6, 2003, www.cnn.com.

"Bezoar." www.themystica.com.

The Centers for Disease Control Web site, www.cdc.gov.

FC&A Medical Publishing, eds., *Natural Cures and Gentle Medicine,* Frank W. Cawood & Associates, 1999.

Goldmann, David R., ed., *The American College of Physicians Complete Home Medical Guide,* DK Publishing, 1999.

Heinrichs, Jay, Heinrichs, Dorothy Belen, and the editors of *Yankee Magazine,* eds., *Home Remedies from the Country Doctor,* Rodale Books, 1999.

"Jenner, Edward," *Encyclopedia Britannica,* 2003, Encyclopedia Britannica

Premium Service, May 23, 2003, www.britannica.com/eb/article?
eu=44512.

Krock, Lexi, "Accidental Discoveries," *Nova Online,* www.pbs.org/
wgbh/nova/cancer/discoveries.html.

Lunia, Dr. P. L., "Sapphire: A Miracle Gem," The Golden India
Foundation Web site, www.indiangyan.com.

"Medicine, History of," *Encyclopedia Britannica,* 2003, Encyclopedia
Britannica Premium Service, May 23, 2003, www.britannica.
com/eb/article?eu=119072.

"Medieval Medical Practitioners," The Mostly Medieval Web site,
www.skell.org.

Mitchell, Rita, "Folk Remedies," The American Medical Association Web site, www.ama-assn.org.

The National Institutes of Health Web site, www.nih.gov.

Physician's Desk Reference for Herbal Remedies, Medical Economics Company, 1998.

Seigworth, Gilbert R., M.D., "Bloodletting Over the Centuries,"
New York State Journal of Medicine, December 1980.

"6 Beauty Lies (and 5 Surprising Truths)," *Cosmopolitan,* August
2002.

Starr, Douglas, "Barber-Surgeons," www.pbs.org.

Thulesius, Olav, "Nicholas Culpepper: English Physician and Astrol-
oger," http://gen.culpepper.com/interesting/medicine/nicholas.
htm.

The 2bnTheWild Web site, http://2bnthewild.com.

The WebMD Web site, www.webmd.com.

The WholehealthMD Web site, www.wholehealthmd.com.

Youngson, Robert M., *Medical Curiosities,* Carroll and Graf, 1997.

CHAPTER THREE

The AFU and Urban Legends Archive, www.urbanlegends.com.

Boughton, Barbara, "Bug Off," The Consumer Health Interactive Web site for Blue Cross and Blue Shield of Minnesota, http://blueprint.bluecrossmn.com/topic/parasitosis.

The Centers for Disease Control and Prevention Web site, www.cdc.gov.

"*Discover* Dialogue: Pathoecologist Karl Reinhard Reconstructing History from the Bottom Up," The *Discover* Web site, www.discover.com/nov_02/breakdialogue.html.

Filer, Joyce M., "Mummy's Ruin? Health Hazards and Cures in Ancient Egypt," The BBC Web site, www.bbc.co.uk/history/ancient/egyptians/health_01.shtml.

Gittleman, Ann Louise, *Guess What Came to Dinner? Parasites and Your Health*, Avery, 2001.

Goldmann, David R., ed., *The American College of Physicians Complete Home Medical Guide*, DK Publishing, 1999.

Illes, Judith, "A Problem as Old as the Pyramids," www.touregypt.net.

"Infection," *Encyclopedia Britannica*, 2003, Encyclopedia Britannica Premium Service, May 24, 2003, www.britannica.com/eb/article?eu=109283.

"It Could Happen to You or Someone You Love," The Bodyfixer Web site, www.bodyfixer.com/parakill.htm.

The Merck Manual of Diagnosis and Therapy, seventeenth edition, on-line edition, www.merck.com/pubs/mmanual.

The National Institutes of Health Web site, www.nih.gov.

"Outbreak of Trichinellosis Associated with Eating Cougar Jerky—Idaho, 1995," The Centers for Disease Control and Prevention "Wonder" Web site, March 15, 1996, http://wonder.cdc.gov.

The *Scientific American* Web site, www.sciam.com.

The Trichinella Web site, www.trichinella.org.

The WebMD Web site, www.webmd.com.

CHAPTER FOUR

"A Collection of Unusual Neurological States," The 23NLPeople Web site, www.23nlpeople.com/Unusual.htm.

"The Cotard Syndrome," The Autism Home Page, http://groups. msn.com/TheAutismHomePage/cotardsyndrome.msnw.

Feldman, Marc D., "Munchausen by Internet: Faking Illness Online," The *Selfhelp Magazine.*Web site, www.selfhelpmagazine.com.

Goldmann, David R., ed., *The American College of Physicians Complete Home Medical Guide,* DK Publishing, 1999.

Howard, Robert, "Folie à Deux Involving a Dog," *American Journal of Psychiatry,* March 1992, vol. 149, no. 3, p. 414.

Idan, Sharon, M.D., and Eliyahu Yona, "Shared Psychotic Disorder," The eMedicine Web site, www.emedicine.com/med/topic3352. htm.

Kasindorf, Martin, "Keeping Manson Behind Bars," *Los Angeles Times,* May 14, 1989.

"Modern Werewolf Cases from Scientific Viewpoints," http:// members.tripod.com/alam25/printer/modern.htm.

Ramsland, Katherine, "All About Stalkers," CourtTV's Crime Library Web site, www.crimelibrary.com.

Ramsland, Katherine, "Factitious Disorders," CourtTV's Crime Library Web site, www.crimelibrary.com.

Shea, John, "The Fragile Orchestra," *The Pennsylvania Gazette,* March 1998, www.upenn.edu/gazette/0398/neuro.html.

Sheldon, David, "The Legend of the Werewolf," The Mystery Database Web site, www.mysterydatabase.com.

"Tourette's Syndrome," *Encyclopedia Britannica*, 2003, Encyclopedia Britannica Premium Service, May 26, 2003, www.britannica. com/eb/article?eu=74966.

Warren, Nick, "Going Through the Looking Glass," *Fortean Times*, April 2001.

The WebMD Web site, www.webmd.com.

The Who Named It? Web site, www.whonamedit.com.

CHAPTER FIVE

"Ambiguous Genitalia," The Medline Plus Medical Encyclopedia, www.nlm.nih.gov/medlineplus/ency/article/003269.htm.

"Aphrodisiacs," The Site Web site, www.thesite.org/magazine/sex_ and_relationships/aphrodisiacs.html.

"Aphrodisiacs: Myth or Magic?" The Improving Sex Web site, www.improvingsex.com/articles/romance/aphrodisiacs.myth.or. magic.htm.

The Armageddon Entertainment Web site, www.armageddon entertainment.com.

"Chief Surgeon to the Weird," *The Sunday Times*, South Africa, December 6, 1998, www.suntimes.co.za/1998/12/06/news/ news35.htm.

"A Collection of Unusual Neurological States," The 23NLPeople Web site, www.23nlpeople.com/Unusual.htm.

"Consumer Information about Viagra," The Food and Drug Administration Web site, www.fda.gov/cder/consumerinfo/viagra/ viagra_consumer.htm.

Diagnostic and Statistical Manual of Mental Disorders, fourth edition, American Psychiatric Association, 1994, text revision, 2000.

The Dictionary of Sexuality Web site, www.sex-dictionary.info/.

Logue, Aaron, "Kluver-Bucy Syndrome," The Library of Neuro-psychological Information Web site, www.loni.com/dands/doc0001.htm.

"Paraphilia," The Discovery.com health Web site, www.health.discovery.com/centers/sex/sexpedia/paraphilia.html.

Pearson, G. A., "Insect Fetish Objects," *Cultural Entymology Digest*, November 1997, www.insects.org/ced4/crush_freaks.html.

"Peyronie's Disease," The National Kidney and Urologic Diseases Information Clearinghouse Web site, www.niddk.nih.gov/health/urolog/pubs/peyronie/peyronie.htm.

"Reproductive System Disease," *Encyclopedia Britannica*, 2003, Encyclopedia Britannica Premium Service, May 26, 2003, www.britannica.com/eb/article?eu=120253.

Tseng, W. S., K. M. Mo, J. Hsu, L. S. Li, L. W. Ou, G. Q. Chen, and D. W. Jiang, "A Sociocultural Study of Koro Epidemics in Guangdong, China," *The American Journal of Psychiatry*, December 1988, vol. 145 no. 12: 1538–43.

Vaughan, "Koro: A Natural History of Penis Panics," www.kuro5hin.org/story/2002/9/16/81843/6555.

"Viewpoints on Asphyxiophilia," www.sexuality.org.

The Vomit Online Web site, www.vomitonline.com.

The World Sex Records Web site, www.world-sex-records.com.

Youngson, Robert M., *Medical Curiosities*, Carroll and Graf, 1997.

Chapter Six

Boone, Allen, "Case Report: Nocturnal Eating Syndrome," *Sleep Review*, www.sleepreviewmag.com.

Brown, Chip, "The Man Who Mistook His Wife for a Deer," *The New York Times*, February 3, 2003.

Butcher, Nancy, *101 Ways to Fall Asleep*, Berkley Books, 2002.

Goldmann, David R., ed., *The American College of Physicians Complete Home Medical Guide*, DK Publishing, 1999.

"Living with Narcolepsy," The National Sleep Foundation Web site, www.sleepfoundation.org/publications/livingnarcolepsy.html.

Mann, Denise, "Bizarre Sleep Disorders," The WebMD Web site, www.webmd.com.

Martin, Lawrence, M.D., "Can Sleepwalking Be a Murder Defense?" www.mtsinai.org/pulmonary/Sleep/sleep-murder.htm.

Schenck, Carlos H., M.D., and Mark W. Mahowald, M.D., "Managing Bizarre Sleep-Related Behavior Disorders," *Postgraduate Medicine*, March 2000, www.postgradmed.com/issues/2000/03_00/schenck.htm.

The Sleepsex Web site, www.sleepsex.org.

Warner, Jennifer, "Gene Linked to Sleepwalking," The WebMD Web site, www.webmd.com.

Webb, Dewey, "Phoenix Babylon, Part 2," *The Phoenix Newtimes* "Mondo Arizona" Web site, www.phoenixnewtimes.com/extra/mondo/mondo3.html.

CHAPTER SEVEN

"Bizarre Tales from A&E," The BBC News Online Web site, http://news.bbc.co.uk/2/low/health/576615.stm.

"Danger in the O.R.? Medical Mistakes Are an Alarming Trend," The ABC News Web site, http://abcnews.go.com/onair/2020/2020_000405_medicalerrors_feature.html.

"Doing His Head In," *Fortean Times*, April 2001 (Associated Press).

"Fly Larvae Grew in Patients at Hospital," *The Saratogian*, March 25, 2002 (Associated Press).

Grady, Dennis, "Oops, Wrong Patient: Journal Takes on Medical Mistakes," *The New York Times,* June 18, 2002.

Inlander, Charles B., Lowell S. Levin, and Ed Weiner, *Medicine on Trial: The Appalling Story of Ineptitude, Malfeasance, Neglect, and Arrogance,* Prentice-Hall Press, 1988.

"The Jester's Courtroom Archive," www.cfif.org/htdocs/legal_issues/ legal_updates/jesters_courtroom/tales_archive.htm.

"Killer Rat," The Weird But True! Web site, www.stephenl.ndtilda. co.uk/page9.htm.

Kirkpatrick, Connie, Ph.D., M.S., R.N., "Safety First: The JCAHO Introduces New Patient Safety Goals," The NurseWeek Web site, www.nurseweek.com.

"Lack of Checks in Kidney Blunder Op," The BBC News Web site, http://news.bbc.co.uk/1/hi/wales/2055752.stm.

"Medical Errors Kill Tens of Thousands Annually, Panel Says," The CNN Web site, www.cnn.com/HEALTH/9911/29/medical. errors/.

Olson, Walter, "A Story That Doesn't Have a Leg to Stand On," *The Wall Street Journal,* March 27, 1995.

"Surgeons' Tools Left Inside 1,500 Patients a Year," the *USA Today* Web site, www.usatoday.com/news/health/2003-01-16-surgical- tools_x.htm.

CHAPTER EIGHT

"Abdominoplasty," The Medical Consumer Guide Web site, www. medicalconsumerguide.com/elective_care/cosmetic_surgery/ abdominoplasty.html.

"Arsenic and Old Telomerase: Hopkins Researchers Unravel Effects of Arsenic on Human Cells." Johns Hopkins Medical Institutions

Office of Communications and Public Affairs Web site, www. hopkinsmedicine.org/press/2001/NOVEMBER/011114.htm.

"Arsenic Poisoning," *Encyclopedia Britannica*, 2003, Encyclopedia Britannica Premium Service, May 26, 2003, www.britannica.com/eb/article?eu=9576.

"Botox for Incontinence," The CBS New York Web site, http://cbsnewyork.com/investigates/local_story_052164115.html.

Bren, Linda, "Saline Breast Implants Stay on Market as Experts Warn About Risks," The Food and Drug Administration Web site, www.fda.gov/fdac/features/2000/400_implant.html.

"Chemical Peels: Surgery Overview," The WebMD Web site, www. webmd.com.

"Do Botox Injections Really Remove Wrinkles?" *The University of California Wellness Letter,*. January 2002.

Garland, Marsha, "Carol Doda and the Topless Era," www.sfnorthbeach.com/g34.html.

Henig, Robin Marantz, "The Price of Perfection," *Civilization Magazine*, April 1996, http://nasw.org/users/robinhenig/price_of_perfection.htm.

"The Jester's Courtroom Archive," www.cfif.org/htdocs/legal_issues/legal_updates/jesters_courtroom/tales_03.html.

King, Victoria, "Arsenic," *History Magazine*, October/November 2000, www.history-magazine.com/arsenic.html.

"Laser Resurfacing: Surgery Overview," The WebMD Web site, www.webmd.com.

"Liposuction: Treatment Overview," The WebMD Web site, www. webmd.com.

The Movie Mistakes Web site, www.movie-mistakes.com.

Stevens, Serita Deborah, with Anne Klarner, *Deadly Doses: A Writer's Guide to Poisons,* Writer's Digest Books, 1990.

"Tattoos and Permanent Makeup," The U.S. Food and Drug Administration's Center for Food Safety and Applied Nutrition Web site, http://vm.cfsan.fda.gov/~dms/cos-204.html.

"Tattoo Problems," The WebMD Web site, www.webmd.com.

"What to Do When You Have a Bellyful," The WebMD Web site, www.webmd.com.

"Woman Dies After Weight-Reducing Surgery," *The Saratogian*, September 10, 2002 (Associated Press).

CHAPTER NINE

The Abiomed Web site, www.abiomed.com.

The Artificial Emotional Creature Web site, www.mel.go.jp/soshiki/robot/biorobo/shibata/aec.html.

"The ASRM Position on Gender Selection," The American Society of Reproductive Medicine Web site, www.asrm.org/Media/Press/genderselection.html.

"Assisted Reproductive Technology," The WebMD Web site, http://my.webmd.com/content/healthwise/8/2084.

The Biopure Web site, www.biopure.com.

Boyles, Salynn, "A Machine to Replace a Failing Heart," The WebMD Web site, http://my.webmd.com/content/article/35/1728_95262.htm.

"Brother and Sister Have Baby to Keep Mother's Fortune," The Ananova Web site, www.ananova.com/news/story/sm_333307.html.

Davis, Lisa, "Miracle Medicine: New Cures, New Fears," *Reader's Digest*, October 2002.

"Gender Selection for Babies Poses Ethical Dilemmas," The CNN Web site, www.cnn.com/HEALTH/9809/09/baby.sex.ethics/.

The Generation 5 Web site, www.generation5.org/aisolutions/jgf-0202.shtml.

"Genomic Tools Identify Profiles of Gene Activity Underlying Cancer," The Duke University Center for Genome Technology Web site, http://mgm.duke.edu/genome/news/tools.htm.

McCarthy, Wil, "Strange Blood," *Wired,* www.wired.com/wired/archive/10.08/blood_pr.html.

The National Institutes of Health Stem Cell Information Web page, http://stemcells.nih.gov/infoCenter/stemCellBasics.asp.

Pollack, Andrew, "Missing Limb? Salamander May Have Answer," *The New York Times,* September 24, 2003.

"62-year-old Woman Gives Birth," The CNN Web site, www.cnn.com/2001/WORLD/europe/05/30/france.mom/.

"65-year-old Indian Woman Becomes the Oldest to Give Birth," The India Express Web site, http://indiaexpress.com/news/health/20030409-1.html.

"Storm Over French IVF Babies," The BBC News Web site, http://news.bbc.co.uk/2/hi/europe/1401070.stm.

Tarquinio, J. Alex, "The Ageless Body," *Reader's Digest,* October 2002.

The WebMD Web site, www.webmd.com.

Index